U0274387

# 温故而知创新

## —— 科研创新经验谈

王秀梅　杜　昶　主编

高等教育出版社·北京

**图书在版编目（CIP）数据**

温故而知创新：科研创新经验谈：中文、英文 /
王秀梅，杜昶主编. -- 北京：高等教育出版社，2016.10
ISBN 978-7-04-046321-7

Ⅰ. ①温… Ⅱ. ①王… ②杜… Ⅲ. ①生物材料-研
究-汉、英 Ⅳ. ①R318.08

中国版本图书馆 CIP 数据核字（2016）第 198133 号

| 策划编辑 | 刘剑波 | 责任编辑 | 卢艳茹 | 封面设计 | 王凌波 | 版式设计 | 张 杰 |
| 责任校对 | 刘春萍 | 责任印制 | 韩 刚 |

| 出版发行 | 高等教育出版社 | | 网 址 | http://www.hep.edu.cn |
| 社 址 | 北京市西城区德外大街4号 | | | http://www.hep.com.cn |
| 邮政编码 | 100120 | | 网上订购 | http://www.hepmall.com.cn |
| 印 刷 | 涿州市星河印刷有限公司 | | | http://www.hepmall.com |
| 开 本 | 787mm×1092mm 1/16 | | | http://www.hepmall.cn |
| 印 张 | 14.25 | | | |
| 字 数 | 240 千字 | | 版 次 | 2016 年 10 月第 1 版 |
| 购书热线 | 010-58581118 | | 印 次 | 2016 年 10 月第 1 次印刷 |
| 咨询电话 | 400-810-0598 | | 定 价 | 69.00 元 |

温故而知创新

李恒绪 2016年2月

業精於勤

柳百新

2016-03-20

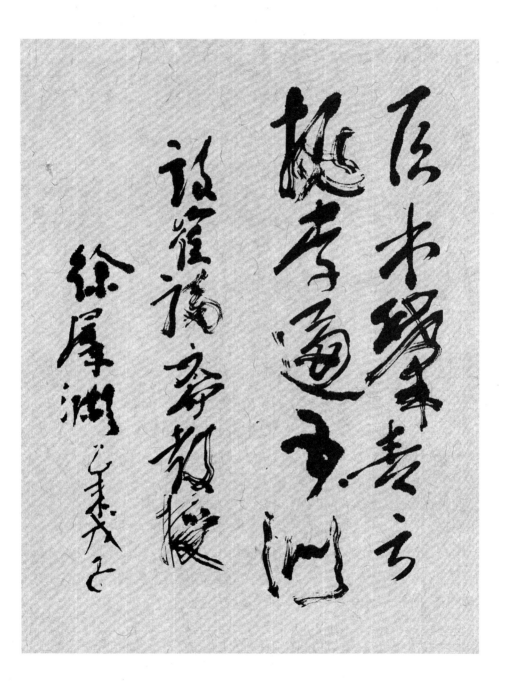

崔福斋教授七十周岁贺

灌溉桃李满天下
创新不止永攀登

山东省立医院
山东省骨科医院
周东生 2016. 六. 11号

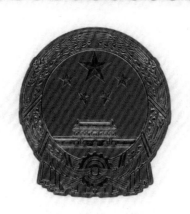

# 国家技术发明奖
# 证 书

　　为表彰国家技术发明奖获得者，特
颁发此证书。

项目名称：纳米晶磷酸钙胶原基骨修复材料

奖励等级：二等

获 奖 者：崔福斋(清华大学)

2008 年 12月 3日

证书号：2008-F-214-2-01-R01

崔福斋教授荣获 2008 年国家技术发明奖二等奖

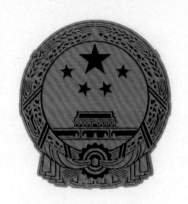

# 国家自然科学奖
# 证　书

为表彰国家自然科学奖获得者，特颁发此证书。

项目名称：生物矿化纤维的分级组装机理研究

奖励等级：二等

获 奖 者：崔福斋(清华大学)

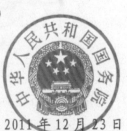

2011 年 12 月 23 日

证书号：2011-Z-108-2-03-R01

崔福斋教授荣获 2011 年国家自然科学奖二等奖

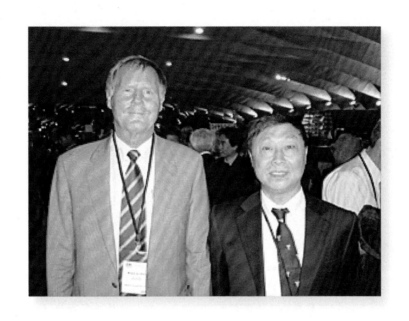

国际材料研究学会联合会授予荷兰 Klaas de Groot 博士及中国崔福斋教授
2003 年度 SOMIYA 奖，奖项名称为《仿生磷酸钙复合材料研究》

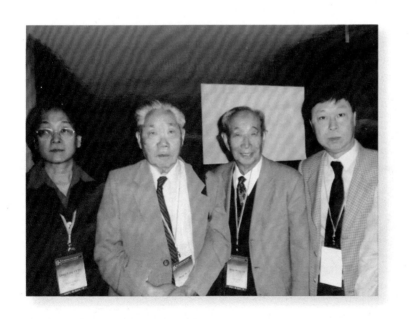

2004 年亚洲生物矿化国际会议上，崔福斋教授做报告后与刘东生院士、
李恒德院士、冯庆玲教授合影

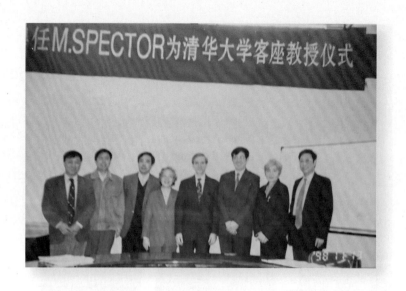

Myron Spector 客座教授聘任仪式上，清华大学副校长关志成教授（右三）、材料学院院长朱静教授（左四）、材料系主任潘伟教授等与聘任建议者崔福斋教授合影

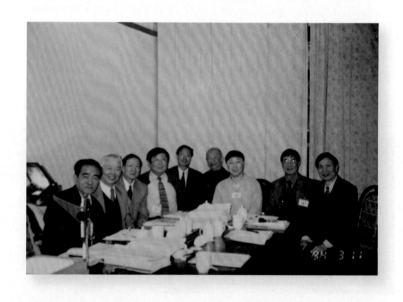

1994 年教育部材料科学重点学科评审委员合影，右一为时任中南大学校长黄伯云，左二为时任华中科技大学校长黄树槐

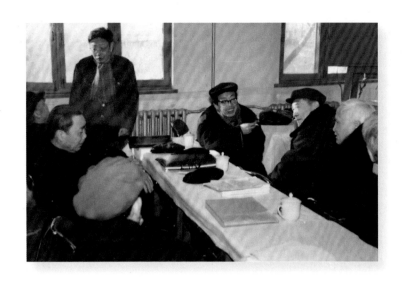

崔福斋博士学位答辩委员会讨论决议，主任为师昌绪先生（右二）

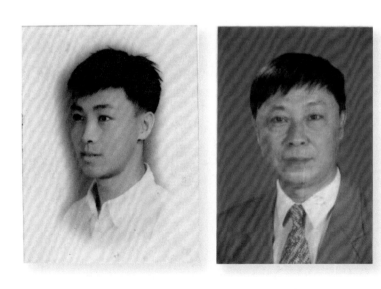

崔福斋教授在清华大学本科一年级时的照片（左）与近年照片（右）

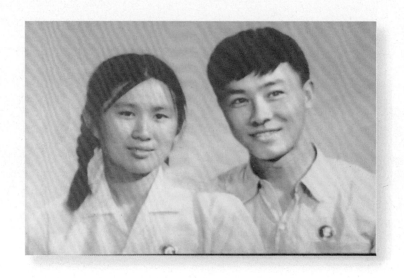

1970 年崔福斋与黄晓兰合影

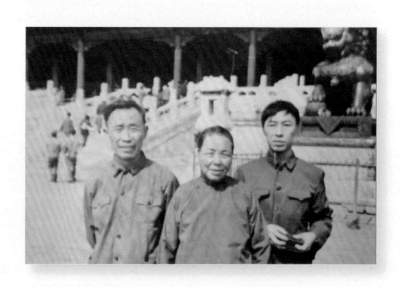

1972 年崔福斋教授带父母游览故宫

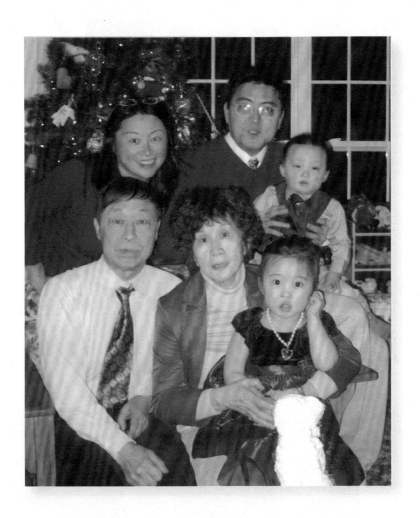

崔福斋教授全家福

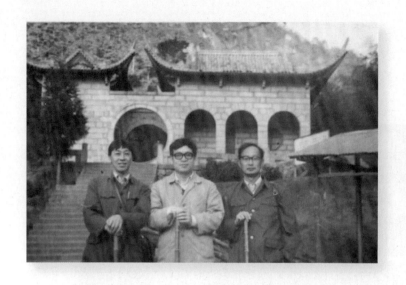

1988 年夏在黄山，参加复旦大学组织的"固体中原子碰撞"国际夏季研讨班的清华大学学员，中间为刚在丹麦获学位回国的顾秉林博士

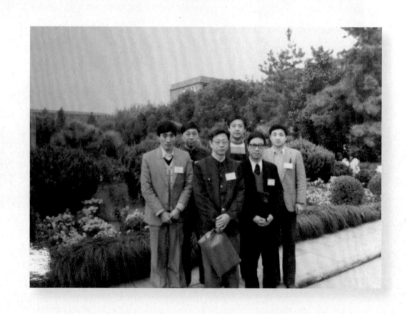

柳百新教授带领清华小组拜访杨福家教授（前排右 1）

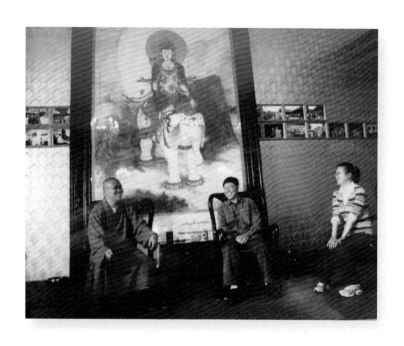

2007 年峨眉山大和尚释永寿与崔福斋教授交谈

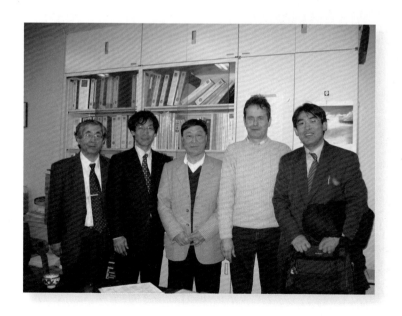

在 Fumio Watari 教授（左1）的办公室，崔福斋教授与几位学者合影

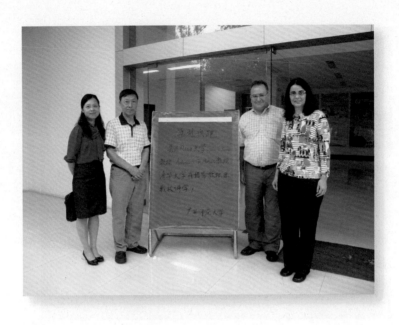

2010 年崔福斋教授陪同 Mikos 夫妇访问广西师范大学

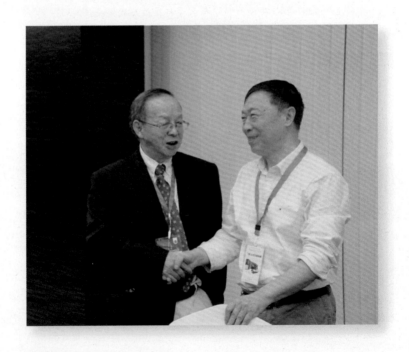

2015 年海口生物材料年会宴会期间，崔福斋教授生日聚会上，张兴栋院士亲来祝贺

# 崔福斋教授博士生毕业答辩照片

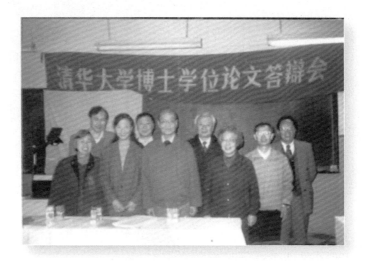

X. W. Su（苏晓维）
- Received Ph. D. degree in 1996
- Postdoctor in CWRU（1997—1999）
- Winner of second class award in the Advancement of Science and Technology from Education Ministry（1998）
- Author of a paper published on *Nature*（1999）
- Research fellow in Cleveland Clinic Center

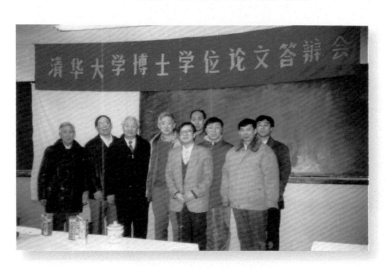

D. J. Li（李德军）
- Received Ph. D. degree in 1998
- Professor of Tianjin Normal University
- Visiting scholar of Northwest University，Chicago

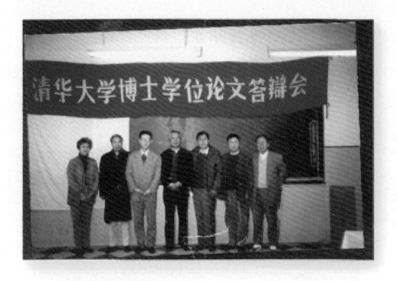

C. Du （杜昶）

- Received Ph. D. degree in 1998
- Winner of Top-Ten graduate students award of Tsinghua University in 1997
- Postdoctor in Leiden University, Holland

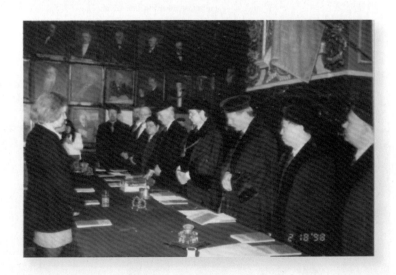

H. B. Wen （温海波）

- Received Ph. D. degree in 1999 （Leiden University）
- Postdoctor in Leiden University, Co-promotion by Klaas de Groot and F. Z. Cui, 1999—2001
- Senior research fellow in DePuy Company from 2001

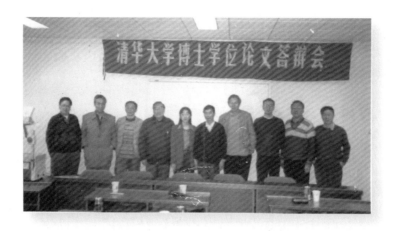

D. M. Zhang（张冬梅）

- Received Ph. D. degree in 1999
- Postdoctor in CWRU （1999—2001）
- Research fellow in Cleveland Clinic Center

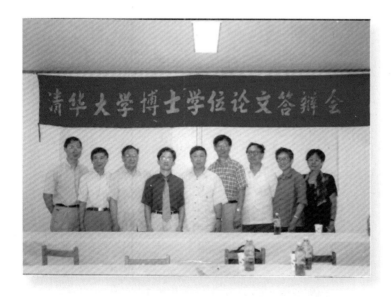

Z. S. Luo（罗忠升）

- Received Ph. D. degree in 2000
- Winner of Top Scholarship of Tsinghua University in 1999
- Winner of excellent Ph. D. thesis of Tsinghua University in 2001
- Visiting scholar at Lawrence Natural Lab

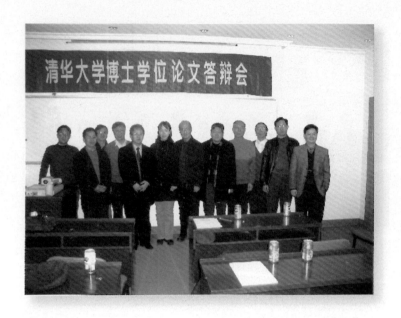

Y. Zhang（张漾）

- Received Ph. D. degree in 2002
- Author of the first paper published in *Bone* from China

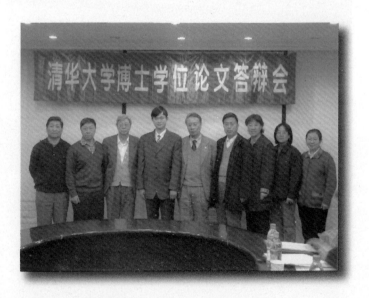

Y. W. Fan（范昱玮）

- Received Ph. D. degree in 2002
- Postdoctor in University of British Columbia
- First Chinese author of paper in *Journal of Neuroscience Methods*

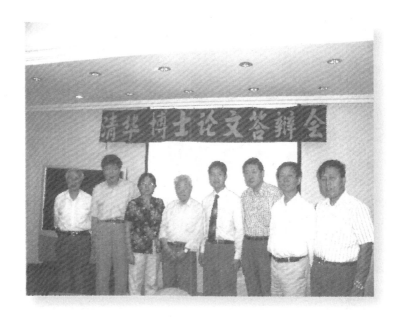

W. Zhang (张伟)

- Received Ph. D. degree in 2004
- Postdoctor in SUNY at Buffalo
- Published a paper in *Chemistry of Materials* which was given a positive note by *Nature Materials*

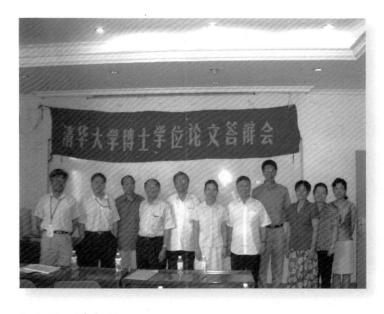

S. S. Liao (廖素三)

- Received Ph. D. in 2003
- First author on *Spine and Tissue Engineering* from China Mainland

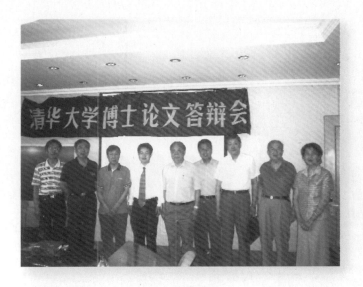

W. M. Tian（田维明）

- Received Ph. D. degree in 2005
- Postdoctor in Medical school of Yale University
- Study on brain tissue engineering scaffold of hyaluronic acid

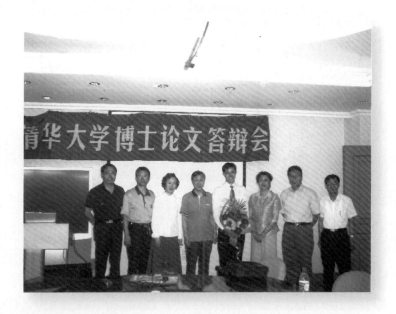

X. D. Kong（孔祥东）

- Received Ph. D. degree in 2005
- Faculty in Life Science College of Zhejiang Sci-Tech University
- Study on biomineralization of silk fibroin by calcium phosphate

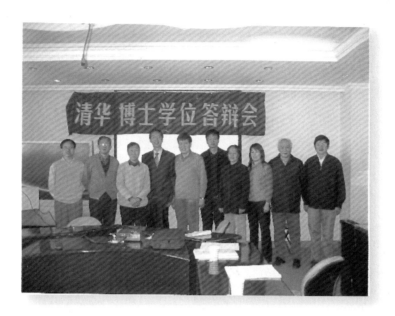

Y. Zhai（翟勇）

- Received Ph. D. degree in 2006
- Study on fibroin structure and two gene materials

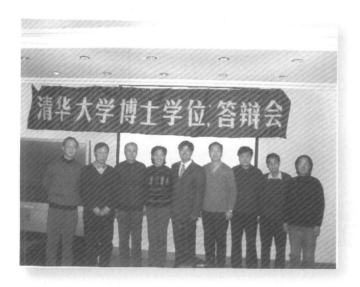

J. Ge（葛俊）

- Received Ph. D. degree in 2006
- New Investigator Award at the Seventh International Symposium on the Composition, Properties and Fundamental Structure of Tooth Enamel（Boston，USA）
- Study on hierarchical structure of enamel and bone and their nanomechanical properties

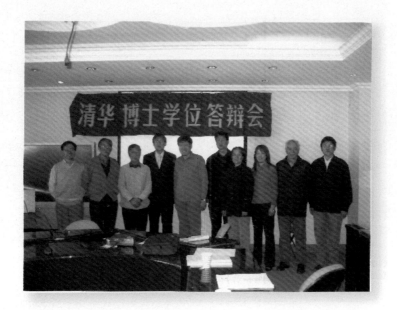

B. Meng（孟波）

- Received Ph. D. degree in 2006
- Study on biodegradable stent materials

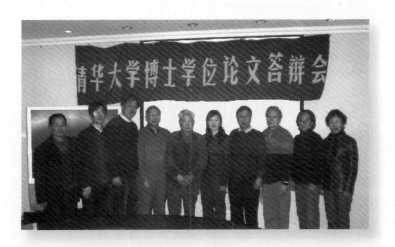

X. M. Wang（王秀梅）

- Received Ph. D. degree in 2004
- Postdoctor in Rochester University
- Established the 7 levels hierarchical structures of zebrafish skeletons; investigated the influences of $liliput^{dtc232}$ gene-mutation on zebrafish bone mineralization

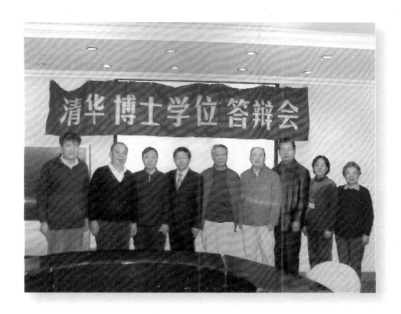

J. Ma（马军）

- Received Ph. D. degree in 2007
- Study on interfacial reaction of neural cells to materials and its related mechanism

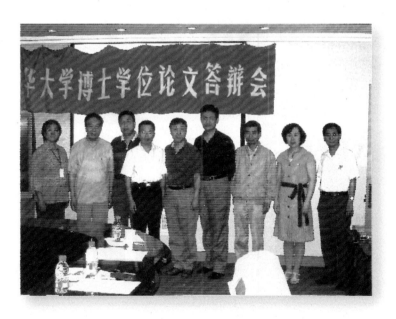

K. Hu（胡堃）

- Received Ph. D. degree in 2007
- Study on recombinant human collagen based biomaterials and its fundamental in vestigation

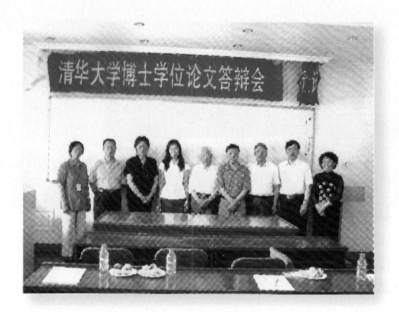

Y. Li（李艳）

- Receive Ph. D. degree in 2008
- Study on the application of bFGF and BMSCs in bone regenerative medicine

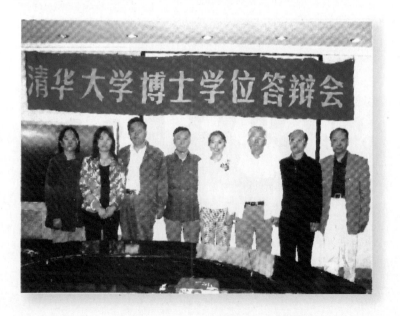

Y. Wang（王玉）

- Receive Ph. D. degree in 2008
- Study on the theory of mineralized collagen formation and the application in bone graft

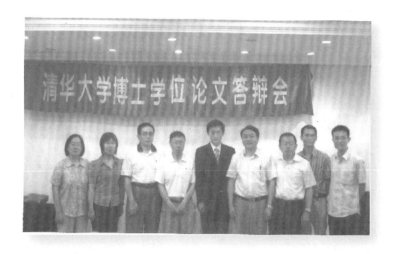

Z. J. Cheng （程振江）

- Received Ph. D. degree in 2010
- Study on protein regulation on biomineralization of bone, teeth and simulation
- Establish the relationships between the gene manipulation and the corresponding alterations on hierarchical structure of bone and enamel

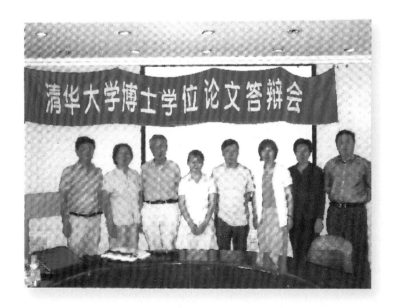

Y. J. Ren （任永娟）

- Received Ph. D. degree in 2009
- Study on regulation of neural stem cells by materials

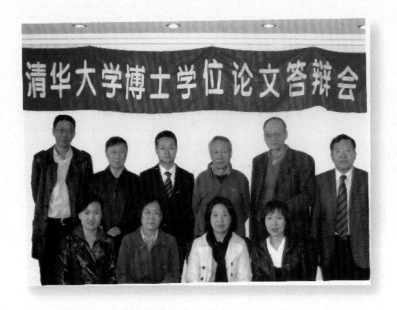

Y. T. Wei (魏岳腾)

- Received Ph. D. degree in 2011
- Study on hyaluronic acid based scaffolds for regeneration of nervous system

# 序

　　当我看到此书稿时，很为崔福斋教授的学生及其合作者的独特思路和奉献精神所感动。他们的想法是，借此机缘，回顾当初合作取得创新性研究成果、发表高被引用文章的经历，分析原因，总结经验；针对生物材料领域如何创新这个永久话题，探讨思路，并展望未来；希望给年轻学者以传统教科书里学不到的理念和参考。我相信，这些经验之谈不仅对生物材料领域的同行有益，也对其他学科的科学工作者有启发。

　　可以自豪地说，中国的生物材料研究经过大家近 30 年来的共同努力，已跻身世界先进水平。这在 2012 年中国召开的世界生物材料大会上，各国生物材料学会代表的评价中已有充分体现。在若干生物材料科学研究方向上，中国的工作处于世界前列已获得国际同行公认，从本书的某些部分也可以看出这一点，例如矿化胶原材料诱导骨组织生长的研究等。

　　我希望，通过本书对"温故而知创新"的探讨，激发大家更多的创意，创造出更多、更好的生物材料与植入器械，为人民健康事业做贡献，并推动科学事业的更大发展。

崔崇栋

2016 年 8 月

# 目　录

# 第一部分

# 崔福斋教授谈科研创新

# 1.1 温故而知创新的实践

崔福斋

创新就是产生新知识或新产品。

知识的定义在认识论中是一个长期争论不止的问题,它激发了世界上众多伟大思想家的兴趣,但至今也没有一个统一而明确的界定。一个经典的定义来自于柏拉图:一条陈述能称得上是知识,必须满足三个条件,它一定是被验证过的、正确的,而且是被人们相信的。

我认为,知识还有两个基本的属性:一是继承性;二是无限性。

要做出创新,就要在无限的未知中发现或造出对人类有益的知识,供继承使用。毫无疑问,谁都希望做出大的创新,对人类做出大的贡献,但是如何做到仍是个问题,对此众说纷纭。

两千多年前,孔子就有"温故而知新"的说法,这应是对这个问题很早期的回答,影响至今。这种回答虽然没有人否定,但太笼统,对初学者不具明确性。因此出现多种注释,不同背景的人理解有所不同。

爱因斯坦与此问题是密切相关的,"提出问题比解决问题更重要"的著名论断广为人知。因为解决问题也许仅仅是一个学术上或实验上的技能而已,但提出新的问题、新的可能性,从新的角度去看旧的问题,却需要有创造性的想象力,而且标志着科学的真正进步。他的这个论断,对有经验的学者有指点迷津的作用,但如何能提出重要的科学问题,特别是基础性问题,可能不是一般学者能做到的。

2015 年中秋节前夕,《中国科学报》记者就如何创新的问题邮件采访了李政道先生。李政道先生在邮件中回答说:"要创新,需学问;只学答,非学问。要创新,需学问;问愈透,创更新。"对于李政道先生的话,我的理解是把爱因斯坦与孔子的话合起来,并深化一步。要做出大的创新,需对前人的知识理解深透,并能提出疑问。

王秀梅教授和杜昶教授提议,在我生日之际邀我的学生及合作者制作一本纪念册。我建议借此机会从各位的成功经验里看看如何具体回答上述问题,集成本书给同行,特别是给年轻人提供参考。同时,各位都是生物材料与组织工程领域的有成就的专家,顺便也展望一下该领域需解决的重要课题,希望能够开发出影响人类生活的创新生物材料。因此,本书起名为《温故而知创新》。

为了抛砖引玉,我愿谈一下自己对"温故而知创新"的体会。

我进入科研领域时，导师是李恒德院士，他给我的课题是关于离子注入改善金属磨损（提高人工关节寿命）的研究。他跟我的初次谈话，我终身不会忘记。

首先，他说这个题目是他从刚参加的国际会议上知道的，是国际关注的课题，并有重要的应用背景。他要求我把该研究课题有关的至少 10 年以来的文献都看完，看别人做到什么地步以及他们的研究特点，还有什么重要问题没有解决，为什么没有解决以及如何解决。李先生还毫无保留地告诉我他的经验。当初，李先生在美国做博士研究时，导师是美国费城宾夕法尼亚大学冶金系 R. M. Brick 教授，Brick 教授一开始就是这样要求他的。Brick 教授是美国当时著名的金属材料科学家。Brick 教授开始给他选择的题目有多个，他经过调研选择研究金属铍的变形机理，这是当时核材料铍加工中急需但未知的科学问题。他的博士论文中的原创工作奠定了人类社会的金属铍机械加工的基础。

李先生得到了富有原创精神的科学家的真传，又传给了他中国的学生。我能成为他第一个博士生，这是很幸运的。这种选题的做法实际与孔子说的"温故而知新"是一致的。

以后我在指导研究生时，也是采取这种套路进行的。我在科研实践中又汲取荷兰的 Klaas de Groot 教授的注重理论的应用、哈佛大学和麻省理工学院的 Myron Spector 教授的注重原始创新、莱斯大学的 Antonie G. Mikos 教授的注重学科交叉、F. Watari 教授的注重实验实践的宝贵经验，为科研创新生涯做到"顶天立地"而积聚了实力。

回想我们之所以能做出较大创新，除上述因素外，还有一个重要条件：我们研究组外部有高水平的国内外合作者，内部始终保持 10 余名博士后、博士生，他们都是优中之优；大家志同道合，以不同学科背景密切合作，多届学生持续深入攻克同一个目标。

我从事科学与工程教学和研究数十年，基本集中在生物材料与组织工程领域，应该说是应用科学领域。这个领域的研究内容应该分为两类，即应用基础研究与产品开发。但无论是选题还是破题，这两类情况都很不同。下面结合自己的经验分别加以叙述。

回顾我和研究生及其他合作者获得的基础性研究成果，主要有：

（1）发现骨骼中矿化胶原多级组装机理。

生物矿化胶原是自然界动物硬组织的基本单元，组成了骨骼、牙齿及其他钙化组织，具有优异的力学性能和生物性能。研究发现，它是有机大分子调制无机矿物沉积得到的基本结构单元，通过自组装实现从纳米尺度到宏观尺度的精确控制和装配，从而形成复杂且高度有序的分级结构。因此，破解矿化胶原多级组装机理是现代生物矿化研究的核心和前沿课题之一。但是长期以来，尽管研究者提出各种模型，尚缺乏矿化胶原多级组装机理的直接证据。

我们详细分析了人骨痂和人胚胎骨样本，并与体外模拟相结合，发现了矿化胶原分级组装机理的三步骤：第一步，单个胶原分子在特定浓度和 pH 条件下，自组装成三股螺旋原胶原纤维；第二步，钙离子和磷酸根离子在胶原特定的羟基和羧基位点结合成核并长大成羟基磷灰石纳米晶，形成矿化胶原微丝；第三步，多根矿化胶原微丝平行结合成矿化胶原纤维簇。

这项成果发表后，在国际上产生了很大影响，*Nature Materials* 专为这项研究发表了评论（附录 1），认为该研究 "给出第一个直接的体外证据，证明了相关的矿化理论"，它 "将提高人类对其他各种矿化组织中胶原调制矿化机理的理解，并为仿生工程制备新型功能材料指明道路"。美国化学学会网站上也发表了署名文章，Jim King 评价该项研究 "发现了关键机理"（附录 2）。美国西北大学 Samuel S. Stupp 教授在 *Chemical Reviews*（IF = 40.2）的综述中用近半页篇幅高度评价了这项科研发现。相关项目《生物矿化纤维的分级组装机理研究》获得了 2011 年国家自然科学奖二等奖（证书编号：2011-Z-108-2-03-R01）。

（2）揭示骨牙分级结构的细微特征。

生物硬组织内部的细致结构如原子排列特征等，至今仍不为人们知晓。而这些未知的关于天然组织的构造原理又是仿生制备生物材料所必须了解的，也是相关学科重要的研究难题。

我们揭示了人体编织骨、斑马鱼脊柱骨、牙釉质、象牙等多种天然矿化组织的分级结构特征，并且为国际学术界认可。牙釉质分级结构模型的提出，推进了人类对牙齿的认识。因此，我被邀请在第 8 届国际生物矿化会议上做大会专题报告。我们因为对象牙多级结构的深入研究，而被邀请为《材料科学技术百科全书》撰写 "lvories" 的条目（附录 3）。另外，人体编织骨的微结构研究结果也广为国内外同行认同，并在研究文献中被大量引用。

（3）生物材料表面改性领域研究有特色。

我们在国际上有特色的研究成果涉及碳氮膜和类金刚石膜与骨细胞、上皮细胞、血细胞、神经细胞以及磷脂的相互作用；钛合金、聚四氟乙烯、聚甲基丙烯酸甲酯和医用镁合金表面镀碳氮膜及类金刚石膜的生物相容性等。镀膜方法涉及离子束沉积技术、磁控溅射技术及其计算机模拟等。因此，近年来，我被邀请在包括美国真空学会 50 周年年会等国际学术会议上做了 5 次学术报告，报告主题包括《碳氮膜或类金刚石膜的生物相容性》等。相关研究获得 1998 年国家教委科技进步奖一等奖。

（4）脑组织工程研究领域的开创者。

我们与神经科学家徐群渊教授合作的关于中枢神经组织工程材料的研究在该领域具有开创性，这是第一次在大脑中植入生物材料并观察到修复效果，被国际刊物 *Biomedical Materials* 评价为 "pioneering the area of brain tissue engineering"（附录 4）。中枢神经的再生是一个世界性的难题，教科书上断言，成熟的中枢神经组织不能再生。本项研究模拟中枢神经组织的细胞外基质的基本成分和结构，探讨以透明质酸为基础的水凝胶作为中枢神经组织工程框架材料的可行性，并通过化学接枝等手段，用防止瘢痕生长的 log66 抗体和多聚赖氨酸等对透明质酸进行改性，显著提高了材料的神经相容性，促进了神经轴突长入，观察到神经再生。同时，我们研究团队在神经干细胞研究领域也取得了创新性的成果：研究了不同化学基团对神经干细胞诱导分化的作用，探索了功能团材料诱导神经再生的机理。在第 8 届世界生物材料大会上，我被选为神经修复材料分会的组织者。

这些科学上的贡献在国际上产生了广泛的学术影响（附录 5~附录 8）。

（5）在技术发明和产品开发方面的主要贡献。

发明了含人骨纳米有序结构的矿化胶原基骨修复材料，并与骨科、神经外科、口腔科医生合作开发了一系列骨修复产品。迄今为止，同类矿化胶原产品美国 FDA（Food and Drug Administration）批准了 6 个，韩国 KFDA（Korea Food and Drug Administration）批准了 1 个，日本 PMDA（Pharmaceuticals and Medical Devices Agency）也批准了 1 个，但他们都没有提到具有人骨的纳米有序结构。

骨组织是人体最重要的组织器官，同时也最容易发生缺损。因此，每年会出现数百万计的骨组织缺损者，他们都需要接受手术治疗。目前的多种骨缺损填充材料皆有各自的局限性。异种骨和异体骨主要存在交叉感染和抗原性的问题；各种以金属、陶瓷或高分子制造的人工骨替代物作为永久植入物，存在着生物相容性差、不能被人体正常吸收等问题；自体骨治疗效果最佳（金标准），但存在着自身供体有限及造成患者额外痛苦等问题。如何在体外制备出在成分和结构上均高度仿生自体骨的骨修复材料是我在进行了大量调研后提炼出的研究课题。

这个问题的解决也是很艰巨的。虽然人体骨骼一直在发育或生长，自组装成复杂有序的骨组织，但是控制自组装的参数组合是未知的奥秘。只有破解这个奥秘，才能实现体外室温自组装类骨材料。我们根据仿生矿化的原理，在体外模拟了骨组织在体内的自组装过程，研制出在分级结构和成分上均与天然骨高度近似的人工骨修复材料。该发明获得美国专利（附录 9）和中国多项发明专利。在材料性能上，它具有优秀的生物相容性、骨传导性以及骨诱导性；在临床使用中，该材料可促进骨组织的重构，诱导新骨形成，并伴随骨缺损修复过程而逐渐降解，无免疫排斥性，无异物残留，治疗效果接近自体骨。

该发明技术的产品已获国家食品药品监督管理总局（China Food and Drug Administration，CFDA）注册证（附录 10），成功实现了临床应用。目前，使用该产品成功治疗的骨缺损患者已经达到 10 余万例，为骨科医生所认可。该产品在 2015 年获美国 FDA 注册证（附录 11），可在世界范围内推广，造福人类。我们的《纳米晶磷酸钙胶原基骨修复材料》项目曾获 2008 年国家技术发明奖二等奖（证书编号：2008-F-214-2-01-R01）。获奖人中包括密切合作的中国人民解放军总医院骨科主任王继芳教授和北京中医药大学东直门医院骨科主任俞兴教授，后者当时刚获得北京大学医学博士学位，到清华大学生物材料实验室做博士后，成功完成第一例矿化胶原骨材料植入人体试验。

（6）医疗器械产品开发的选择。

其实关于医疗器械产品开发的选题，换句话说，就是选择什么产品进行开发，那就不单是科学问题，还要考虑一系列社会学因素。全国生物材料教授、研究员近千人，但有开发生物材料植入物医疗器械产品经验者寥寥无几，因此，交流这个对我国特别重要的论题显得尤其必要。

例如，当初的冠状动脉支架产品的选题就很成功。该产品开发出来后，每年拯救数百万人的生命，同时，每年也创造出近千亿的产值。当然，其发明者与进行产品化的并不是同一个人。后来模仿者的开发是另一个话题。

技术发明或产品模型有很多，如何选择好的医疗器械产品去开发，当然也是一种选题问题（目的是为社会服务的同时公司获得最大的利润），但这是一门系统的学问，论述起来需要说很多话。鉴于这个问题特别重要，我有正反两方面的经验，也听过跨国公司首席技术官的经验之谈。我的见解概述如下：

第一，考虑该产品市场的大小。医院用量越大，越值得开发。

第二，考虑该产品技术含量的大小，知识产权明确。确定适应症有无其他产品，如有，那么确定该产品的技术原理是否比原有产品的技术原理先进，治疗效果是否更好，产品技术有无技术诀窍，是否容易仿制。

第三，考虑该产品售价与生产成本的比例。可接受的售价是客观存在的，成本越低，利润越高。

第四，考虑投产和获得产品注册证的难易程度。投产周期越长，临床试验费用越大；办证需时越长，费用越高。

第五，考虑该产品市场推广的难易程度，包括是否容易使用。这涉及销售成本的大小。

第六，考虑该产品单件价格的高低。过高的单价是不利因素。

企业在有多项产品需要选择时，通常应该权衡这六大因素。如果第一考虑最佳为 10 分，从第二考虑开始依次递减 1 分，第六考虑满分为 5 分，那么对几项产品打分后，选最高分的产品进行开发应是明智的选择。

最后，依据本人对生物材料与组织工程学科和无源医疗器械行业的了解与思考，提出 10 年后若干重要科研课题和重要新产品展望如下，仅供讨论与思考：

（1）寻找材料因素对人体免疫系统影响的主要规律。

（2）材料因素（基因组）引起干细胞（以及癌细胞）分化的规律性研究。

（3）关于从厘米到纳米的分级结构研究深入到人体若干组织，包括 DNA。

（4）破译天然生物材料编码自组装过程细节研究。

（5）中枢神经（脊髓、脑组织）修复与再生研究。

（6）生物材料药物复合体用于癌症治疗研究。

（7）带神经和毛发的皮肤组织工程研究。

（8）带生物牙根的牙种植体普及。

（9）带多生长因子的矿化胶原基骨修复产品普及。

（10）微创手术配合植入物手术普及，取代一半以上传统开放手术。

（11）材料复合干细胞产品批准进入临床试验。

（12）心脑血管全降解支架产品普及。

（13）体外合成矿化胶原密质骨。

# 1.2 崔福斋教授主要科研成绩及评价

## 1.2.1 代表性文章/著作

1. Zhang W, Liao S S, Cui F Z. Hierarchical self-assembly of nano-fibrils in mineralized collagen. *Chemistry of Materials*, 2003, 15 (16): 3221-3226.

　　该研究探索并提出了矿化胶原的组装过程及机理, *Nature Materials* (Vol. 2, 2003, p. 566) 专为这项研究发表了评论, 给予了高度评价。SCI 引用 230 次。

2. Cui F Z, Li D J. A review of investigations on biocompatibility of diamond-like carbon and carbon nitride films. *Surface and Coatings Technology*, 2000, 131 (1-3): 481-487.

　　首次在碳氮膜合成中采用 $NH_3$ 方法制备出高性能碳氮膜, 并在生物材料中进行应用。SCI 引用 235 次。

3. Du C, Cui F Z, Zhu X D, de Groot K. Three-dimensional nano-HAp/collagen matrix loading with osteogenic cells in organ culture. *Journal of Biomedical Materials Research*, 1999, 44 (4): 407-415.

　　该研究的主要贡献在于设计实验, 发现矿化胶原与骨细胞的作用机理。SCI 引用 248 次。

4. Fan Y W, Cui F Z, Hou S P, Xu Q Y, Chen L N, Lee I S. Culture of neural cells on silicon wafers with nano-scale surface topograph. *Journal of Neuroscience Methods*, 2002, 120 (1): 17-23.

　　该研究找到了适合神经细胞在材料表面生存的最佳表面光洁度。SCI 引用 142 次。

5. Du C, Cui F Z, Zhang W, Feng Q L, Zhu X D, de Groot K. Formation of calcium phosphate/collagen composites through mineralization of collagen matrix. *Journal of Biomedical Materials Research*, 2000, 50 (4): 518-527.

　　该研究的主要贡献在于报导了三维矿化胶原材料的形成机理及细节。SCI 引用 188 次。

6. Du C, Cui F Z, Feng Q L, Zhu X D, de Groot K. Tissue response to nano-hydroxyapatite/collagen composite implants in marrow cavity. *Journal of Biomedical Materials Research*, 1999, 42 (4): 540-548.

该研究的主要贡献在于报导了三维矿化胶原材料与成骨细胞的反应规律。SCI 引用 166 次。

7. Liao S S，Cui F Z，Zhang W，Feng Q L. Hierarchically biomimetic bone scaffold materials：Nano-HA/collagen/PLA composite. *Journal of Biomedical Materials Research Part B：Applied Biomaterials*，2004，69B（2）：158-165.

该研究的主要贡献是完成了发明材料体内骨修复特征检测。SCI 引用 228 次。

8. Du C，Su X W，Cui F Z，Zhu X D. Morphological behaviour of osteoblasts on diamond-like carbon coating and amorphous C–N film in organ culture. *Biomaterials*，1998，19（7-9）：651-658.

国际上首次报导了碳氮膜和骨细胞的反应特征。SCI 引用 97 次。

9. Kong X D，Cui F Z，Wang X M，Zhang M，Zhang W. Silk fibroin regulated mineralization of hydroxyapatite nanocrystals. *Journal of Crystal Growth*，2004，270（1-2）：197-202.

国际上首次报导了丝素蛋白调制羟基磷灰石的矿化。SCI 引用 84 次。

10. Tian W M，Hou S P，Ma J，Zhang C L，Xu Q Y，Lee I S，Li H D，Spector M，Cui F Z. Hyaluronic acid-poly-D-lysine-based three-dimensional hydrogel for traumatic brain Injury. *Tissue Engineering*，2005，11（3-4）：513-525.

我国最早开展透明质酸脑组织工程研究的团队之一。SCI 引用 99 次。

11. Ren Y J，Zhang H，Huang H，Wang X M，Zhou Z Y，Cui F Z，An Y H. In vitro behavior of neural stem cells in response to different chemical functional groups. *Biomaterials*，2008，30（6）：1036-1044.

报导了化学功能团调控神经干细胞分化的规律。SCI 引用 73 次。

12. Xu S J，Qiu Z Y，Wu J J，Kong X D，Weng X S，Cui F Z，Wang X M. Osteogenic differentiation gene expression profiling of hMSCs on hydroxyapatite and mineralized collagen. *Tissue Engineering Part A*，2015，22（1-2）：170-181.

首次证实了仿生矿化胶原比羟基磷灰石具有更高的成骨活性。

13. 崔福斋，冯庆玲. 生物材料学. 北京：科学出版社，第一版，1996；北京：清华大学出版社，第二版，2004.

14. 崔福斋，生物矿化. 北京：清华大学出版社，第一版，2007；第二版，2012.

15. *Encyclopedia of Biomedical Engineering*. Editor：Metin Akay，Wiley，2006，Article 1403：Tissue Engineered Bone：3545-3549.

16. *Encyclopedia of Materials：Science and Technology*. Editor：George D W Smith，Elsevier，2001，Article：Ivories：4327-4329.

# 1.2.2 发明专利

1. 发明人：Cui F Z，Zhang S M，Zhang W，Cai Q，Feng Q L；专利名称：Nano-calcium phosphates/collagen based bone substitute materials；批准年份：2005 年；专利号：US 6887488 B2.

美国发明专利，该项专利的研究成果是一种结构和成分高度仿生的纳米晶磷酸钙胶原基骨修复材料，已经在临床上广泛应用。该项专利为获得美国 FDA 认证提供了条件，同时也为开拓海外市场奠定了基础。

2. 发明人：崔福斋，张曙明，廖素三，冯庆玲，李恒德；专利名称：纳米相钙磷盐/胶原/高分子骨复合多孔材料的制备方法；批准年份：2001；专利号：ZL 01129699. 2.

本项发明介绍了一种用于骨修复领域的纳米相钙磷盐/胶原/高分子骨复合材料的制备方法，制备出的材料在结构与成分上具有仿骨性。获得 2006 年国家知识产权局中国专利优秀奖。

3. 发明人：崔福斋，蔡强，张曙明；专利名称：纳米相钙磷盐/胶原/聚乳酸骨复合多孔材料的制备方法；批准年份：2003；专利号：ZL 00107493. 8.

本项发明提供了一种用于骨修复的纳米相钙磷盐/胶原/聚乳酸多孔材料的制备方法，制备出的材料具有大量的连通微孔，与人体松质骨结构相当。此专利被北京奥精医药科技有限公司购买，独家投资 100 万。

4. 发明人：崔福斋，张曙明，廖素三，冯庆玲；专利名称：含有纳米相钙磷盐、胶原和海藻酸盐的骨材料的制备方法；批准年份：2004；专利号：ZL 01141901. 6.

本项发明涉及了一种含有纳米相钙磷盐、胶原和海藻酸盐的骨材料的制备方法。此材料的生物相容性好，强度和孔隙率适当，可以作为植入型可降解骨材料而得到应用。

5. 发明人：崔福斋，罗忠升，冯庆玲；专利名称：医用植入物的离子束增强沉积羟基磷灰石镀层的制备方法；批准年份：2000；专利号：ZL 97120353. 9.

本项发明提供了一种医用植入物的离子束增强沉积羟基磷灰石镀层的制备方法。本发明制备的镀层具有膜与基片的结合力强、膜本身致密度高、生物相容性优良等优点。

6. 发明人：崔福斋，孔祥东，张敏；专利名称：矿化丝蛋白材料及其制备方法；批准年份：2006；专利号：ZL 200410003453. 6.

本项发明涉及一种矿化丝蛋白材料及其制备方法，该材料可应用于生物医用材料领域，其矿化物为钙磷盐纳米晶体。该材料具有良好的生物相容性和骨诱导性。

7. 发明人：崔福斋；专利名称：含 bFGF 胶原基纳米人工骨及其制备方法；批准年份：2008；专利号：ZL 200810052950.3.

本项发明介绍了一种含 bFGF 胶原基纳米人工骨及其制备方法，所载 bF-GF 可从载体上持续缓慢释放，缓释期至少 10 天，提高载体骨修复材料的成骨活性，提高胶原基纳米人工骨的临床效果。

8. 发明人：崔福斋，田维明，徐群渊，侯少平，魏岳腾；专利名称：一种中枢神经修复用水凝胶材料及其制备方法；批准年份：2006；专利号：ZL 200610011425.4.

本发明涉及一种水凝胶材料，具有与中枢神经组织相近的流变学特性和力学性能，植入中枢神经以后不会对组织造成二次伤害，制备方法简单，成本低，适合大规模生产。

9. 发明人：崔福斋，范俊，冯庆玲，崔凯；专利名称：一种用于引导组织再生的复合膜制备方法；批准年份：2005；专利号：ZL 03150163.X.

本发明提供了一种用于引导组织再生的纳米晶羟基磷灰石/胶原/聚乳酸-羟基乙酸复合膜材料的制备方法。材料具有一个表面粗糙、另一个表面光滑的结构特点，其降解速率、膜厚度和膜的力学性能均可实现调节控制。

10. 发明人：崔福斋，田维明，张存理，俞兴，董何彦；专利名称：用于手术后防粘连的带药加铁离子的透明质酸凝胶；批准年份：2006；专利号：ZL 03133843.7.

本发明所制备的防粘连剂在体内存留时间长，可有效预防外科手术后粘连，在体内可自行降解，无需手术取出，降解产物对人体无害。

11. 发明人：仇志烨，王昶明，崔福斋；专利名称：矿化胶原复合骨粘合及填充材料；批准年份：2015；专利号：ZL 201410040803.X.

## 1.2.3　重要科技奖项情况

1. 获奖人姓名：崔福斋，王秀梅，李恒德，蔡强，孔祥东；获奖项目名称：生物矿化纤维的分级组装机理研究；2011 年；国家自然科学奖；二等奖（一等奖空缺）.

阐明生物硬组织结构单元——生物矿化纤维的分级组装机理，为发展新型组织工程支架材料提供新思路。

2. 获奖人姓名：崔福斋，冯庆玲，李恒德，王继芳，俞兴，蔡强；获奖项目名称：纳米晶磷酸钙胶原基骨修复材料；2008 年；国家技术发明奖；二等奖.

该成果主要用于骨缺损患者的骨修复治疗，在牙科修复以及美容整形领域也有广阔的应用前景。目前，临床应用成功治愈骨缺损患者两万余例，效果接近自体骨。

3. 获奖人姓名：崔福斋，Klaas de Groot；获奖项目名称：仿生磷酸钙复合材料研究；2003 年；国际材料研究学会联合会颁发；SOMIYA 奖（每年一项）．

4. 获奖人姓名：李恒德，崔福斋，冯庆玲；获奖项目名称：磷酸钙系生物矿物及其仿生制备；2003 年；教育部提名国家科学技术进步奖；二等奖．

    该成果首次在体外情况下模拟了磷酸钙体系生物矿化过程，采用自组装方法制备纳米晶羟基磷灰石/胶原复合材料，开拓了国际上仿生自组装制造医用材料的新途径。

5. 获奖人姓名：崔福斋，范毓殿，李恒德；获奖项目名称：载能束材料科学的若干研究基础；1999 年；教育部科技进步奖；二等奖．

6. 获奖人姓名：崔福斋，冯庆玲，李恒德，王继芳，蔡强；获奖项目名称：纳米晶磷酸钙胶原基骨修复材料；2006 年；国家教委科技进步奖；一等奖．

    该项科研成果模拟体内生物矿化原理，制备出在结构和成分上高度仿生的骨移植替代材料。该产品已经在全国大面积推广，同时也在向国际推广。

7. 获奖人姓名：柳百新，李恒德，崔福斋；获奖项目名称：载能离子束与金属相作用的基础研究；1988 年；国家教委科技进步奖；一等奖．

    该项科研成果主要是多元靶中原子碰撞级联模拟及动态靶模拟的计算模型。

8. 获奖人姓名：崔福斋，张曙明，廖素三，冯庆玲，李恒德；获奖项目名称：纳米相钙磷盐/胶原/高分子骨复合材料多孔材料的制备方法；2006 年；中国专利奖；中国专利优秀奖．

    该成果提供了一种结构高度仿生的骨修复材料的制备方法，该材料可以广泛应用到颈椎病、腰椎病、拔牙创、骨缺损等领域，临床反馈无一例有毒副作用和不良反应。

9. 获奖人姓名：付伟军，崔福斋等；获奖项目名称：组织工程尿道支架重建战创伤后尿道的研究；2010 年；军队科技进步奖；二等奖．

10. 获奖人姓名：安沂华，崔福斋等；获奖项目名称：干细胞-组织工程学技术修复周围神经损伤的实验研究；2011 年；武警部队科技进步奖；二等奖．

# 附　　　录

## 附录 1　*Nature Materials* 评论（图片通过 Copyright Clearance Center 获得许可使用）

### RESEARCH NOTES

#### Switching liquid crystals with light

Organic photochromes — molecules that can be converted between two isomeric forms by light irradiation — have potential applications in rewritable optical memories and photonic switches. However, for optical memory applications, the organic materials must be stable under repeated writing and readout processes, and should have excellent fatigue resistance. Glassy materials, which can be easily processed into large-area films without grain boundaries, offer significant advantages in this respect. Shaw H. Chen and colleagues at the University of Rochester have reported in *Advanced Materials* (15, 1061–1065; 2003) the first morphologically stable photoresponsive glassy liquid crystals. The materials consist of a photochromic diarylathene core functionalized with nematogens, resulting in a monodomain glassy nematic film. Irradiation of the film with ultraviolet light converts the photoresponsive core molecules from an open-ring form to a closed-ring form, in which the electronic transition moment is aligned with the nematic director. This photochromic reaction results in a large refractive index change. The researchers hope to improve the photoresponsive properties of the material by increasing the degree of uniaxial alignment of the liquid crystalline films.

#### Simultaneous bioassays

A more sophisticated tool for analysing blood that measures not only the glucose level but also the insulin concentration would help in the therapeutic management of diabetes. Moreover, it may facilitate the diagnosis of pancreatic malfunction and insulinoma, a tumour that produces excess insulin. This capability could soon become available through the combination of the enzymatic assay for glucose, and the immunological assay for insulin, in a microfluidic chip built by a group of researchers at the New Mexico State University (*Journal of the American Chemical Society* 125, 8444–8445; 2003). Through a judicious sequence of reactions and electrophoretic separation, the two different assays can be conducted simultaneously on the same blood droplet and without any interference problems, despite the two substances under analysis differing hugely in concentration (millimolar for glucose and nanomolar for insulin). Whether or not this particular chip will actually be used for the management of insulin-related diseases is hard to predict. But it definitely shows the possibility of combining bioassays based on distinct assay principles in a miniaturized analyser.

#### Ultrasensitive real-time sensing

Individual nanoscale particles are particularly attractive as platforms for *in vivo* sensing of chemical species and monitoring of dynamic processes inside biological cells. They have several advantages over traditional sensing approaches, such as their small size — making them non-invasive — and improved sensitivity. Richard Van Duyne and Adam McFarland at Northwestern University, writing in *Nano Letters* (http://dx.doi.org/10.1021/nl034372s), describe the use of dark-field optical microscopy to demonstrate the optical response of single silver nanoparticles to the adsorption of a monolayer of around 100 zeptomoles ($100 \times 10^{-21}$ moles) of small organic molecules. This suggests that the limit of detection for a single nanoparticle is well below 1,000 molecules for small-molecule adsorbates. The sensing principle relies on the electronic sensitivity of the noble-metal surface states to local changes in dielectric constant induced by the adsorbates. The kinetics of the nanoparticle response was also investigated and shown to be comparable to the kinetics of other real-time sensor technologies.

#### Synthetic bone

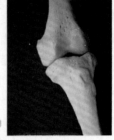

Animal tissues such as bone and muscle are composed of a hierarchical assembly of nanofibrils and mineralized collagen, which allows these specialized tissues to perform different functions. Zhang and colleagues in Beijing have now prepared these nanofibrils synthetically to form a structure and composition that resembles that of bone (*Chemistry of Materials* 15, 3221–3226; 2003). They took different compositions of monomeric collagen and solutions containing calcium and phosphate ions, then used either pH or temperature to induce the formation of collagen fibrils. Transmission electron microscopy at both low and high resolution revealed the different levels of organization. The authors found that nanocrystals of the minerals were deposited along the surface of the fibrils — giving the first direct evidence to support previous theories that this occurs. The authors suggest that the growth of the crystals is controlled by the fibrils themselves, in that the c axes of the crystals align themselves along the longitudinal axes of the fibrils. The mineralized fibrils then align parallel to each other to form fibres. These results should improve the understanding of collagen-mediated mineralization in other calcified tissues, and point the way to new functional materials for biomimetic engineering.

#### POLISHING WITHOUT CRACKING

As you might expect, diamond films used in optical applications have to be extremely uniform. Diamond has many advantages over conventional optical coatings, such as optical transparency at many wavelengths, resistance to wear and even biocompatibility, which makes it especially useful in microfluidic devices. Owing to their exceptional hardness, however, diamond films are not easy to modify following deposition — micromachining usually results in cracking or peeling. In the August issue of the *Review of Scientific Instruments* (74, 3889–3892; 2003) Yongqi Fu and colleagues in Singapore offer a solution. Diamond films deposited by standard CVD processes were subjected to focused ion-beam milling with gallium ions, and were found to retain their optical and chemical properties. With this technique the authors etched a diffractive optical element, involving six concentric rings, directly into the surface of a diamond film. The diffraction efficiency of this optical element was 73%, which is acceptable for most applications.

#### Chemical logic

You might call it physics-envy. Since the 1950s chemists have been trying to recreate solid-state circuits and devices using electrochemical systems. The first electrochemical cells that could amplify, rectify and integrate signals were called solions. In the 1980s, researchers used microelectrode arrays coated with conducting polymers to mimic some functions of diodes and field-effect transistors. In the *Journal of the American Chemical Society* (http://dx.doi.org/10.1021/ja0366585), Wei Zhan and Richard Crooks report the first successful diodes and transistors based on microfluidic electrochemical systems. Their devices consist of indium tin oxide electrodes patterned onto glass, and crisscrossed by microscale channels embedded in a polymer mould. When solutions containing electrolytes or other reagents flow through the channels, diode-like or transistor-like behaviour is observed. The authors use the same approach to construct optoelectronic devices, the most complex of which has seven electrodes and operates as a NAND gate.

566

nature materials | VOL 2 | SEPTEMBER 2003 | www.nature.com/naturematerials

© 2003 Nature Publishing Group

14

# 附录 2 美国化学学会网站评价（图片经美国化学学会许可使用）

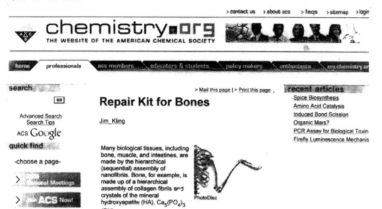

> contact us　> about acs　> faqs　> sitemap　> login

## chemistry.org
### THE WEBSITE OF THE AMERICAN CHEMICAL SOCIETY

home　professionals　acs members　educators & students　policy makers　enthusiasts　my.chemistry.or

search

Advanced Search
Search Tips
ACS Google

quick find
-choose a page-

> ...tional Meetings
> ACS Now!

> ACS Membership Benefits
> CEN-CHEMJOBS

> Mail this page | > Print this page

## Repair Kit for Bones

Jim_Kling

Many biological tissues, including bone, muscle, and intestines, are made by the hierarchical (sequential) assembly of nanofibrils. Bone, for example, is made up of a hierarchical assembly of collagen fibrils and crystals of the mineral hydroxyapatite (HA), $Ca_5(PO_4)_3(OH)$.

PhotoDisc

The most important factor in building bone tissue is the proper alignment of HA crystals with collagen. Studies have shown that this alignment may be directed by anionic groups on the surface of collagen interacting with calcium cations in HA. However, this hypothesis remains uncertain because no one has characterized the hierarchical assembly of mineralized collagen nanofibrils.

In an upcoming issue of Chemistry of Materials, W. Zhang, S. S. Liao, and F. Z. Cui of Tsinghua University (Beijing) describe how they used conventional and high-resolution transmission electron spectroscopy (HRTEM) to study nanofibrils of mineralized collagen [ASAP, DOI: 10.1021/cm030080g]. They have found a key mechanism behind how these fibrils self-assemble, and the results of their study could apply to bone formation. They also demonstrate for the first time that HA crystals associate specifically with the surfaces of collagen fibrils.

The researchers focused on a specific mineralized fiber and found that hierarchical assembly occurs in three stages. In the first, collagen molecules self-assemble into triple helices, forming fibrils about 5 nm wide. HA crystals then associate with the fibrils in the second stage, with their axes orienting along the long axes of the collagen fibrils. This implies that the collagen fibrils have a strong influence on the growth of the crystals. The diameters of the mineralized fibrils are between 5.5 and 6.9 nm. In the third stage, the mineralized collagen fibrils line up parallel to one another to form mineralized collagen fibers 77 to 192 nm wide.

The HRTEM analysis is the first direct evidence that the HA phase is polycrystalline (composed of many small crystals) and forms a layer that covers the surface of the collagen fibrils.

The observation that the crystals align themselves with the long axis of the collagen fibrils is important. Previously, researchers had found that anions on the collagen molecules act as nucleation sites for HA crystals and that the positions of the hydroxyl groups in HA crystals lie along the same axis as the carbonyl groups in collagen. This finding suggests that the two functional groups are responsible for the alignment, perhaps through a dual interaction with HA's calcium cations.

This nanoscale organization mirrors that seen in HA crystals in mineralized tissues, further suggesting that this knowledge could be useful in the design of new materials for bone tissue repair. A deeper understanding of how these materials form could be a boon to materials scientists as they attempt to make other functional materials, such as scaffolds for bone growth that could be absorbed by the body.

This article first appeared on August 4, 2003.

附录 3 崔福斋研究团队因为对象牙多级结构的深入研究，而被邀请为《材料科学技术百科全书》撰写 "Ivories" 的条目（图片通过 Copyright Clearance Center 获得许可使用）

## Ivories

Ivories are a variety of hard, dense, smooth, usually cream-colored materials that include the tusks or the upper incisors of elephants and other mammals such as hippopotamus, walrus, narwhal, sperm whale, and some types of wild boar and warthog. There is another kind of ivory, namely vegetable ivory, which is obtained from the ivory nut, the seed of a South American palm. The ivory commonly used in commerce comes from the dentin part of the tusk of elephants. Both the African elephant and the Indian elephant have tusks, but the female Indian elephant may have smaller tusks or none at all. Ivory is prized for its beauty, elasticity, durability, and suitability for carving figurines, other art objects, and other articles such as billiard balls and the keys of a piano. In the past, most commercial ivory came from the African elephant (*Loxodonta africana*), the number of which rapidly declined to the point of extinction during the twentieth century. In order to save the African elephant from extinction, the trade and hunting of ivory are banned by the Convention on Trade in Endangered Species (CITES). Hence substitute materials have been developed to meet the unrelenting demand for ivory. Since the mid-1950s, natural ivory has been largely replaced by artificial materials. Furthermore, the attractive properties of ivory have aroused interest in studying the structure and the structure–function relation in ivory. In the following section, the composition, properties, and hierarchical structure of ivory are described in detail.

### 1. The Composition of Ivory

Ivory is composed of 30 wt.% organic matter and 70 wt.% minerals. The main component of the organic matter is a complex network of type I collagen fibers, which are rich in proline and glycine (Miles 1967, Linde 1984, Raubenheimer *et al.* 1990). The minerals in ivory are hydroxyapatite (HA), where some of the $Ca^{2+}$ ions (about 18%) in the h.c.p. (hexagonal close packed) crystal lattice of HA ($Ca_{10}(PO_4)_6(OH)_2$) are substituted by $Mg^{2+}$ ions with an average atomic concentration ratios of Ca:Mg:P = 1.3:0.4:1.0 (Zhang *et al.* 1991). There are a total of 20 elements in the inorganic fraction of ivory, and 17 amino acids in the organic fraction (Raubenheimer *et al.* 1998). The composition varies geographically by region, and it has been reported that ivory from African elephants has a higher mineral content than that of Indian elephants (Rajaram 1986, Raubenheimer *et al.* 1998). The variation can be utilized to identify the source of the original ivory (Raubenheimer *et al.* 1998).

### 2. Properties of Ivory

Ivory is durable, incombustible and suffers little by immersion in water; it has a density near $1.7 \times 10^3 \, kg\,m^{-3}$ and can be polished beautifully. Moreover, it works well with woodworking tools.

Compared with mammalian compact bone samples, ivory requires greater work to fracture but has a lower tensile strength and modulus. Examination of wet ivory from Indian elephants showed that the average tensile strength, elastic modulus, and work to fracture of ivory were $36\,MN\,m^{-2}$, $3.5\,GN\,m^{-2}$, and $4.9 \times 10^{-5}\,J\,m^{-2}$, respectively, compared with $99.2\,MN\,m^{-2}$, $17.7\,GN\,m^{-2}$, and $4.0 \times 10^{-5}\,J\,m^{-2}$ for bovine femur (Rajaram 1986).

Ivory has a hardness comparable to lamellar bone. Under a load of 50–200 g, the Vickers microhardness of ivory was determined to be 0.30–0.45 GPa. Anisotropy of mechanical propertics was observed in the natural ivory. Among three orthogonal planes related to the cylindrical geometry of the tusk, the circumferential plane is the hardest plane while the radial plane is the softest one. The mechanical discrepancy may come from the special fabric reinforcement structure organized with preferential orientations of collagen fibers and mineral crystals. (Cui *et al.* 1994).

### 3. The Structural Hierarchy of Ivory

Figure 1 illustrates the hierarchical structure of ivory. A characteristic "chequer-board" pattern was shown on the polished transverse plane (Raubenheimer *et al.* 1990). The pattern is made up of two sets of radially distributed layers of collagen fibril bundles, which interweave into a network. Each of the layer has a thickness of 0.3–0.5 mm. Within a layer, the fibril bundles of 2 μm in diameter remain nearly parallel to one another and oblique to the transverse plane of the tusk. They rotate by about 90° from one layer to the next. The bundles of collagen fibrils are composed of dense-packed mineralized collagen fibrils, 60–200 nm in diameter. These collagen fibrils are packed approximately longitudinally along the main axis of tusk, while the nanocrystallites of HA predominantly deposit in the gap zones of the packed fibrils (Su and Cui 1999).

All crystals in ivory are plate shaped with an average size of 38 [001] × 20 × 3–5 nm, which are much smaller than crystals in bone (50 × 25 × 1.5–4 nm). The smaller crystal sizes in ivory may account for the lower mineralization and may further contribute to their lower strength and modulus, which allow ivory to be easily shaped into pieces of art (Cui *et al.* 1994).

The apatite crystals in ivory are distributed both within the collagen fibrils and in the extrafibrillar space. The amount of apatite crystals deposited within the collagen fibrils and in the extrafibular spaces is 65% and 35%, respectively. The apatite crystals in the collagen fibrils are predominantly distributed within the gap zone of the collagen fibrils, with [001]

1

16

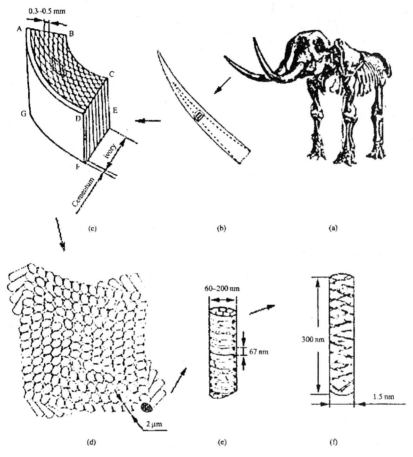

**Figure 1**
The hierarchical structure of ivory. (a) An elephant skeleton showing the development of the upper incisors (tusks). (b) The interior hollow cavity of a tusk. (c) Enlargement of a block of tusk showing the "chequer-board" pattern on the transverse plane and two layer of the tusk on the radial plane: the coating layer of 1–2 mm in thickness is cementum; the interior of the tusk is ivory (transverse plane, plane ABCD; radial plane, plane DCEF; circumferential plane, plane ADFG). (d) Enlargement of the rhombic region marked by the dashed line in (c) showing the array pattern of mineralized collagen bundles, each bundle depicted as a cylinder composed of several tens to several hundreds of collagen fibrils as shown in (e) with minerals deposited mainly in their gap regions (e) A single collagen fibril with a 67 nm band feature. (f) A triple-helical molecule of collagen.

preferential orientation parallel to the axial direction of the collagen fiber or the main axis of the tusk. Differently, the crystals in the extrafibrillar spaces are stacked along the tangential plane of the collagen fibrils, with their long axes parallel to the collagen fibrils. The distribution of minerals is thought to arise

2

17

from the variation of the organic matrix for calcification. The proteins in the extrafibrillar space are noncollageneous, where apatite crystals fill in the voids to stabilize the structure of the collagen fibrils and increase the integrity of the whole structure, thereby reinforcing the mechanical properties of ivory (Su and Cui 1997).

## 4. Summary

Ivory is a biological material with a high economic value that is used extensively for carved figurines and other objects of art. It is a biocomposite organized with collagen fibrils and mineral crystals at hierarchical levels, from nanometers up to millimeters. At the primary level, ivory is structurally identical to other collagen composite systems such as dentin and bone, where collagen molecules composed of amino acid chains align longitudinally in a quarter-staggered pattern to form gap zones that are filled by plate-shaped crystals. At higher levels the ivory is organized notably as two sets of radially distributed layers of collagen bundles which interweave to form a network matrix, where each of the bundles are parallel to one another within the same layer and rotated by approximately 90° from one layer to its neighbor. The unique properties of ivory result from this specific construction. However, investigations to date of the structure and properties of ivory have yet to match the hierarchical structure to the properties at each level of organization.

## Bibliography

Cui F Z, Wen H B, Zhang H B, Li H D. Liu D C 1994 Anisotropic indentation morphology and hardness of natural ivory. *Mater. Sci. Eng.* **C2**, 87–91
Linde A 1984 Ultrastructure of dentin and dentinogenesis. In: *Dentin and Dentinogenesis*. CRC press, Boca Raton, Vol. 1, p. 81
Miles A E W 1967 Microanatomy and histochemistry of dentin. In: *Structural and Chemical Organization of Teeth*. Academy Press, New York, Vol. 2, p. 3
Rajaram A 1986 Tensile properties and fracture of ivory. *J. Mater. Sci. Lett.* **5**, 1077–80
Raubenheimer E J, Brown J M M, Rama D B K, Dreyer M J, Smith P D, Dauth J 1998 Geographic variations in the composition of ivory of the African elephant (*Loxodonta africana*). *Arch. Oral Biol.* **43**, 641–7
Raubenheimer E J, Dauth J, Dreyer M J, Smith P D, Turner M L 1990 Composition and structure of the ivory of the African elephant. *S. Afr. J. Sci.* **86**, 192–3
Su X W, Cui F Z 1997 Direct observations on apatite crystals in ivory. *J. Mater. Sci. Lett.* **16**, 1198–200
Su X W, Cui F Z 1999 Hierarchial structure of ivory: from nanometer to centimeter. *Mater. Sci. Eng.* **C7**, 19–29
Zhang H B, Cui F Z, Wang S, Li H D 1991 Characterizing hierarchial structure of natural ivory. *Mater. Res. Soc. Symp. Proc.* **255**, 151

F. Z. Cui

Encyclopedia of Materials: Science and Technology
ISBN: 0-08-0431526
pp. 4327–4329

3

附录 4　被国际刊物 *Biomedical Materials* 评价为"pionee-ring the area of brain tissue engineering"（图片通过 Copy-right Clearance Center 获得许可使用）

IOP PUBLISHING                                                                                     BIOMEDICAL MATERIALS

Biomed. Mater. 5 (2010) 060201 (2pp)                                              doi:10.1088/1748-6041/5/6/060201

## EDITORIAL

# Fu-Zhai Cui's vision and leadership

**Editors-in-Chief**

**In-Seop Lee**
*Yonsei University, Seoul,
Korea*

**Myron Spector**
*Harvard Medical School, VA
Boston Healthcare System,
MA, USA*

Our colleague and friend, Fu-Zhai Cui, has decided to step down from his position as Co-Editor-in-Chief of *Biomedical materials* (BMM) at the end of the year due to other commitments.

BMM would not be the journal that it is, and we two would not have served as participants in its development, were it not for Fu-Zhai. It was his vision and hard work that gave birth to BMM. Fu-Zhai's e-mail to Dr Mingfang Lu at IOP Publishing in June of 2005 initiated the process that led to the new journal being established. Underscoring the importance of such an endeavor, Fu-Zhai noted that biomedical materials and tissue engineering and their applications had been rapidly developing in recent years and the trend was likely to continue for many years, that there were relatively few journals capable of handling these subjects, and even fewer journals that faced East as well as West.

There are several features of Fu-Zhai's professional life which have added to the character of BMM and which reflect, and perhaps even help to explain, his country's remarkable development: resourcefulness, innovation, and drive. When we first met Fu-Zhai at Tsinghua University more than 15 years ago, the facilities available to him were notably limited, especially in comparison to those that we had access to at our respective institutions. There was almost a complete absence of biomaterials-related journals at Tsinghua, prompting us to consider ways in which we could send our surplus issues to him. But Fu-Zhai made the most of what resources he did have and directed his students in important and productive research that was published in leading English-language journals. Fu-Zhai never let his thinking and efforts be constrained by limited resources.

The projects undertaken by Fu-Zhai and his students at Tsinghua have always displayed engineering innovation born of scientific understanding. He is either investigating biomaterials for new applications or taking novel approaches for the production of new types of biomaterials. In both cases, his work is founded on knowledge drawn from an array of scientific studies and his success is due in large part to the multidisciplinary teams that he assembles. For example, Fu-Zhai's group was one of the first in the world to employ biomaterial implants (hyaluronic acid hydrogels) for the treatment of brain defects, thus pioneering the area of brain tissue engineering. For other biomaterials applications, such as bone tissue engineering, Fu-Zhai took the biomimetic approach of producing mineralized collagen scaffolds. But he did so in the novel way of co-precipitating collagen and hydroxyapatite to favor self-assembly and a hierarchical microstructure. Fu-Zhai's insights into the mineralization process were derived in part from his own studies with Heng-De Li, one of the pioneers of biomineralization.

Biomaterials researchers frequently think about the potential clinical applications of their developments, but rarely find or make the opportunity to commercialize their products. Fu-Zhai acted on translational research before that term entered the researcher's lexicon. He orchestrated the compilation of pre-clinical data and engaged his clinical colleagues in the necessary human trials to demonstrate the safety and efficacy of his mineralized collagen scaffolds for spine fusion and other applications. After having been approved by the China medical device regulatory process, the product is now being used in clinics.

1748-6041/10/060201+02$30.00                                                                1

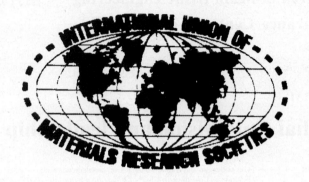

# IUMRS

# 2003 SOMIYA AWARD

## for

### International Collaborative Research

*FuZhai Cui*

R.P.H. Chang, IUMRS General Secretary & Founding President

附录 6　至 2016 年 3 月初，SCI 关于崔福斋的文章发表及引用数据

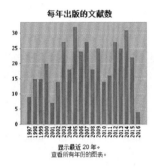

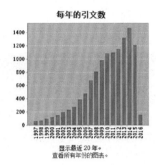

| | |
|---|---|
| 找到的结果数: | 436 |
| 被引频次总计[?]: | 12342 |
| 去除自引的被引频次总计[?]: | 11388 |
| 施引文献 [?]: | 9269 |
| 去除自引的施引文献[?]: | 8991 |
| 每项平均引用次数[?]: | 28.31 |
| h-index [?]: | 55 |

附录 7　Science 关于中国组织工程的报道，多处提及崔福斋的工作（图片通过 Copyright Clearance Center 获得许可使用）

Biomaterials

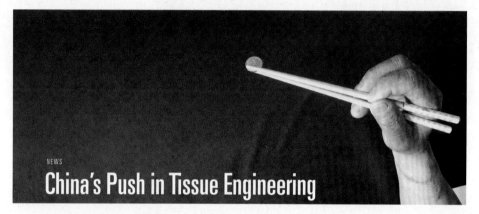

NEWS

# China's Push in Tissue Engineering

Valued for their innovation potential, biomaterials efforts in China prosper

sudden onset of funding. When Spector revisited the Tsinghua professor's lab a few years later, he was shocked at the improvement in available resources and science being conducted. He listened in awe as Cui's graduate students described innovative biomaterials they were developing to treat defects in the brain resulting from conditions such as stroke. "I had just never heard anything like it," Spector recalls. "I thought, 'This is really out there.'"

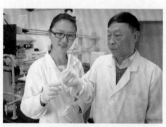

**Bone doctor.** Cui Fuzhai (*right*) developed a bone repair scaffold that has been used by 30,000 patients.

length, location, and diameter," says Yang Xiongli, a neuroscientist at Fudan University in Shanghai.

Gu was also the first to translate this artificial nerve research to the clinic. China's State Food and Drug Administration (SFDA) gave approval for clinical trials in 2010. A trial is now under way at four Chinese hospitals, with 35 grafts completed. Gu expects that it will conclude next year.

He's also combining his chitosan-based its application is being pursued elsewhere in the world, he says.

Translational research promises to become one of China's strengths in tissue engineering, says Cao, the plastic surgeon whose work on cartilage engineering originally helped spark interest in the field. Now director of the Shanghai Key Laboratory of Tissue Engineering, he and Liu are working on clinical applications of engineered cartilage, bone, tendon, skin, and blood vessel grafts.

But the regulatory hurdles can still be substantial in China. Individual components of the grafting process require safety approvals before any clinical trials can start. Thus, Cao and Liu have yet to receive SFDA

major grant programs, 863 and 973, as well as from the National Natural Science Foundation of China. The 973 Program focuses on basic research, and from 2009 to 2011, its funding for nanotechnology, a category that encompasses advanced materials, advanced diagnostics, electronics, and tissue engineering, totaled more than $82 million, according to Lux Research. From 2006 to 2011, the Program poured $77 million into tissue en neering and stem cell research.

entists on how to navigate the trial application process and steer their research toward the clinic. "The important thing is China now has the funding mechanisms, both public and private, and the SFDA is now acting judiciously," Spector says. But it could take time before more scientists achieve the success that Gu has had in moving their research into the clinic. "The central government has put a lot of money into this field," says Dai, who mentored some of China's younger tissue engineering researchers and remembers when things were very different. "The problem has become how to use it—so we don't waste it."

**–MARA HVISTENDAHL**

Published by AAAS

22

附录 8　由于崔福斋教授在生物材料，特别是生物矿化纤维组装机理方面的影响力，2007 年被美国医学与生物工程学院（American Institute for Medical and Biological Engineering）选举为 Fellow；因骨修复材料的卓著研究成果，2008 年被国际生物材料科学与工程学会联合会（International Union of Societies for Biomaterials Science and Engineering）选举为 Fellow

AMERICAN INSTITUTE FOR MEDICAL AND BIOLOGICAL ENGINEERING

In recognition of outstanding contributions to the field of
Medical and Biological Engineering

*Fu-Zhai Cui, Ph.D.*

Has been elected a Fellow of the Institute.

March 2007

Chairman, College of Fellows

President, AIMBE

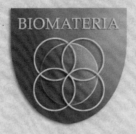

*Be It Known That*

# FUZHAI CUI

*has been duly elected to*

*Fellow, Biomaterials Science and Engineering*

# FBSE

*Attested on this 28th day of May in the year 2008*

YOUNG HA KIM, PRESIDENT
INTERNATIONAL UNION OF SOCIETIES FOR BIOMATERIALS SCIENCE & ENGINEERING

# 附录9　人工骨修复材料获得美国专利

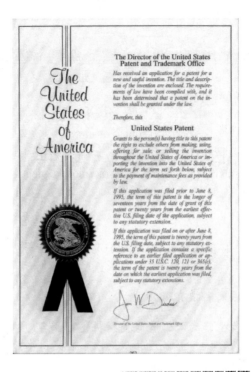

(12) **United States Patent**　　　　(10) Patent No.: **US 6,887,488 B2**
Cui et al.　　　　　　　　　　　　　(45) Date of Patent:　　　**May 3, 2005**

US006887488B2

(54) **NANO-CALCIUM PHOSPHATES/COLLAGEN BASED BONE SUBSTITUTE MATERIALS**

(75) Inventors: **Fuzhai Cui**, Beijing (CN); **Shuming Zhang**, Beijing (CN); **Wei Zhang**, Beijing (CN); **Qiang Cai**, Beijing (CN); **Qingling Feng**, Beijing (CN)

(73) Assignee: **Tsinghua University**, Beijing (CN)

( * ) Notice: Subject to any disclaimer, the term of this patent is extended or adjusted under 35 U.S.C. 154(b) by 390 days.

(21) Appl. No.: **09/845,724**

(22) Filed: **May 2, 2001**

(65) **Prior Publication Data**

US 2002/0018797 A1 Feb. 14, 2002

(30) **Foreign Application Priority Data**

May 19, 2000　(CN) ......................... 00107493

(51) Int. Cl.⁷ ......................... **A61F 2/00**; C12N 11/14; C12N 11/02; C12N 5/06; C12N 5/08

(52) U.S. Cl. ......................... **424/426**; 424/93.7; 435/176; 435/177; 435/395

(58) Field of Search ........................... 424/426, 93.7; 435/176, 177, 395

(56) **References Cited**

U.S. PATENT DOCUMENTS

| | | | |
|---|---|---|---|
| 5,626,861 A | 5/1997 | Laurencin et al | 424/426 |
| 6,013,591 A | 1/2000 | Ying et al. | 501/1 |
| 6,331,312 B1 | * 12/2001 | Lee et al. | 424/426 |

FOREIGN PATENT DOCUMENTS

WO　　WO 00/03747　　1/2000

* cited by examiner

*Primary Examiner*—David M. Naff
(74) *Attorney, Agent, or Firm*—Crowell & Moring LLP

(57)　　**ABSTRACT**

The present invention relates to a nano-calcium phosphates/collagen composite that mimics the natural bone, both in composition and microstructure, as well as porous bone substitute and tissue engineering scaffolds made by a complex of said composite and poly(lactic acid)(PLA) or poly (lactic acid-co-glycolic acid)(PLGA). The invention also relates to the use of said scaffold in treating bone defect and bone fracture.

**10 Claims, 2 Drawing Sheets**

# 附录 10 人工骨修复材料获得 CFDA 产品注册证

## 中华人民共和国
### PEOPLE'S REPUBLIC OF CHINA

## 医疗器械注册证
### REGISTRATION CERTIFICATE FOR MEDICAL DEVICE

注册号： 国食药监械(准)字2014第3461579号

北京奥精医药科技有限公司：

你单位生产的人工骨修复材料（商品名：骼金），经审查，符合医疗器械产品市场准入规定，准许注册。自批准之日起有效期至二零一九年九月四日。

特此证明。

国家食品药品监督管理总局
China Food and Drug Administration
2014 年注册专用章 日

附件：医疗器械注册登记表

No.1406680

# 附录 11 人工骨修复材料（Bongold）于 2015 年获美国 FDA 注册证

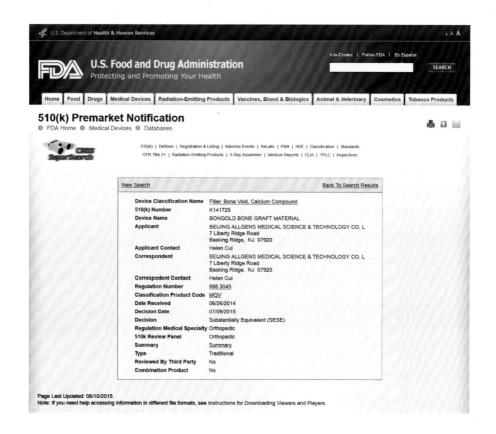

# 第二部分

# 国内外合作者忆谈创新

# 2.1 In Honor of Dr. Fu-Zhai Cui's 70th Birthday

Esther J. Lee and Antonio G. Mikos

Rice University, Houston, TX, USA

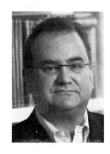

Antonio G. Mikos，世界著名的生物材料专家。美国莱斯大学生物工程与化学、生物分子工程教授，该校生物医学工程 J. W. Cox 实验室和组织工程"卓越中心"主任。美国国家工程院和医学科学院两院院士。国际著名 SCI 收录期刊 *Tissue Engineering*（*Part A*，*Part B*，*Part C*）的创始编辑及主编。国际组织工程与再生医学学会（Tissue Engineering and Regenerative Medicine International Society，TERMIS）的 Founding Fellow。曾担任 TERMIS 美国学会主席，美国生物材料学会（SFB）主席。

We heartily congratulate Dr. Fu-Zhai Cui on his prolific scientific career as a leader and visionary in the field of biomaterials at this milestone of his 70th birthday. May the coming years abound with further inspiration and discovery, advancing the work for which the foundation has already been laid.

Dr. Cui embarked on his undergraduate and graduate education at Tsinghua University, then traveled abroad for a two-year postdoctoral position at FOM (Fundamental Research on Matter) Institute for Molecular and Atomic Physics in Amsterdam, the Netherlands. He eventually returned to his alma mater, joining the faculty of Tsinghua University in the Materials Science and Engineering department in 1992 and subsequently rising to the rank of Professor of Biomaterials Science and Director of the Institute for Regenerative Medical and Biomimetic Materials. As a testament to his productive academic career thus far, he has authored over 400 publications and mentored many successful students throughout this period.

Moreover, he has exercised outstanding leadership as Editor-in-Chief of *Biomedical Materials*, in addition to actively participating on the editorial board of *Journal of*

*Materials Science: Materials in Medicine*, *Journal of Bioactive and Compatible Polymers*, *Journal of Tissue Engineering and Regenerative Medicine*, *Tissue Engineering*, and *Journal of the Royal Society: Interface*. Dr. Cui has also placed tremendous value on disseminating scientific knowledge in this age of global research by organizing various conferences, including the 6th World Biomaterials Congress and the 10th International Symposium on Biomineralization. For these collective contributions, he has been recognized with numerous awards in China and received the prestigious honor of being elected as a fellow to the American Institute for Medical and Biological Engineering and the International Union of Societies for Biomaterials Science and Engineering.

Over the course of his research career, Dr. Cui has explored many avenues, demonstrating the breadth and depth of his knowledge as a leading authority in biomaterials and tissue engineering. He has contributed an extensive body of work regarding the characterization and application of materials. Dr. Cui has studied the utility of calcium phosphate coatings to enhance osseointegration at the implant-bone interface. Most importantly, he pioneered hydroxyapatite/collagen materials for bone tissue engineering applications. His earlier work showed that hydroxyapatite crystal formation resulted from carboxylate and amino groups present on collagen, which bound to calcium and phosphate, respectively. More recently, Dr. Cui has developed injectable bone fillers consisting of mineralized collagen and calcium sulfate hemihydrate, which may have tremendous potential as minimally invasive materials for repair.

As a leading authority in tissue engineering, Dr. Cui has successfully fostered numerous academic collaborations worldwide. Together with him, I (AGM) and other colleagues evaluated the responses of bone marrow and adipose tissue sourced mesenchymal stem cells when maintained under different encapsulation strategies in collagen and synthetic hydrogels. Our study revealed that cell proliferation and osteogenesis were indeed influenced by hydrogel type and loading method (Ma et al., *Journal of Biomedical Materials Research Part A*, 2014). In addition, Dr. Cui and I have surveyed the viewpoints of leading scientific leaders following the 5th Aegean Conference on Tissue Engineering in Kos, Greece. We disseminated their diverse insights on what they envision for the future of the field for the benefit of current researchers and emerging scholars (Cui and Mikos, *Regenerative Biomaterials*, 2014). Indeed, the impact of Dr. Cui's scientific inquiries extends beyond the laboratory. His longstanding focus on purposefully developing clinically translatable technologies has flourished in the form of issued patents in China and the United States. Most prominently, Dr. Cui has developed nano-calcium phosphate and collagen hybrid scaffolds possessing structural properties reminiscent of native bone for repairing related defects and traumatic fractures. The utility of such implants has additionally been specified for spinal fusion applications. Aside from acquiring patents, Dr. Cui has played an instrumental role in transforming these mineralized collagen composites into products marketed by the Beijing Allgens Medical Science & Technology Company, which have craniofacial, dental, and orthopedic applications.

I (EJL) had the honor of meeting Dr. Cui at the 5th Aegean Conference on Tissue Engineering in Kos, Greece in June 2014. His creativity, vision, and passion for science were evident when showcasing his research endeavors, and as a graduate student in the early stage of my scientific career, I was able to gain new perspective on bone tissue engineering strategies employing mineralized collagen composites.

I (AGM) have had the pleasure of knowing Dr. Cui as friend and colleague for over 20 years. We have enjoyed fruitful academic collaborations, and I look forward to seeing the ongoing successes of this research partnership.

Dr. Cui has made many outstanding contributions as a researcher, mentor, and leader in tissue engineering, and we wish him all the best as he continues to pursue his academic passions and inspire the next generation of scientists!

# 2.2 Memories of My Collaboration with Prof. Cui

Klaas de Groot

ACTA Department of Oral Implantology and Prosthetic Dentistry,
University of Amsterdam, The Netherlands

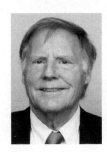

Klaas de Groot，荷兰阿姆斯特丹大学教授，生物陶瓷专家。培养出 40 余名生物材料博士，其中 16 名来自中国大陆，与崔福斋教授联合培养了温海波医学博士及杜昶医学博士。曾获国务院总理颁发的友谊勋章，2010 年获美国生物材料学会 Clemenson 论文奖。2005 年欧洲生物材料学会主席。

Let me start with congratulating Prof. Cui, a worldwide respected scientific colleague, with his 70th birthday. We met more than 20 years ago, and soon thereafter we felt the need to initiate joint scientific projects between his group at Tsinghua University in Beijing and my group, then at Leiden University, in Leiden, The Netherlands, and our first scientific publication appeared in 1997. Prof. Cui visited our country already much earlier: after finishing his undergraduate and graduate education at Tsinghua University, he traveled abroad for a two-year postdoctoral position at FOM Institute for Molecular and Atomic Physics in Amsterdam, the Netherlands. So, it might have been the case that he and I unwittingly met somewhere in Amsterdam far before our biomaterials research cooperation started!

But back in China he changed his field of interest from theoretical physics to biomaterials. Joining the faculty of Tsinghua University in 1992 he subsequently rose to the rank of Professor of Biomaterials Science and Director of the Institute for Regenerative Medical and Biomimetic Materials. And he did well: his more than 400 publications and the many successful students he supervised are a testament to his exceptional academic career. In addition, he achieved numerous international awards. As I intend to focus on our scientific joint venture, I will not dwell on his participation in editorial boards, in organizing conferences, in getting awards, and more in general his involvement in disseminating scientific knowledge worldwide, but more on "what we did together".

Except for one award we jointly received: the Japanese SOMIYA Award. From the website of the SOMIYA Award we can read that the fourth time this award was presented (in the year 2003) Prof. Cui and myself were the joint recipients and based on our joint research on "Biomimetic Calcium Phosphate Composites" (Award Location: Yokohama, Japan).

I think the titles of the work of two students of his Tsinghua group who successfully defended their Ph. D. thesis at our Biomaterials Research Group at Leiden University says it all: Hai-Bo Wen got his Dutch Ph. D. degree with his thesis "Calcium phosphate coatings based on mineralization in natural hard tissues" on February 18, 1998, and a few years later (December 18, 2002) Chang Du received his Ph. D. degree with the thesis entitled "Biomimetic composites for bone substitution". The truly international nature of our cooperation was emphasized by the Leiden University appointment of Prof. Cui as guest-supervisor besides me as the Leiden University supervisor.

Dr. Hai-Bo Wen studied the utility of calcium phosphate coatings to enhance osseointegration at the implant-bone interface. Actually, in doing so, he positioned himself as one of the grandfathers of what is now known as Biomimetic CaP coatings, a room temperature method to coat dental and orthopedic implants. It must please Prof. Cui, that almost twenty years later the institution where I am currently connected with, namely ACTA (Academisch Centrum Tandheelkunde Amsterdam), received a 2 million Euro grant to conduct a clinical trial, in preparation for a FDA approval, of biomimetically coated dental implants. The Dutch industry CAM Bioceramics plans to produce such implants in the near future.

Dr. Chang Du pioneered hydroxyapatite/collagen materials for bone tissue engineering applications, based on earlier work of Prof. Cui showing that hydroxyapatite crystal formation resulted from carboxylate and amino groups present on collagen, which bound to calcium and phosphate, respectively. As the results of our joint scientific inquiry on collagen calcium phosphate composites ultimately extend beyond our laboratories into products marketed by the Beijing Allgens Medical Science & Technology Company, which have craniofacial, dental, and orthopedic applications, we conclude that not only Dutch industry profits from our collaboration, but Chinese as well.

How about our joint students themselves? Did they profit from our Dutch-China cooperation? I think the answer is an unequivocally "yes". Dr Hai-Bo Wen currently holds the important position of Director of Dental Research of one of the largest biomedical companies in the world, namely Zimmer Biomet, and is located in the USA, while Dr Chang Du got a position as a professor of Biomedical Engineering at South China University of Technology. With already more than 60 publications and a RG (ResearchGate) score of 33, he is becoming one of the leading biomaterial scientists of China, and indeed of the world.

I am sure that I not only speak for myself but also for my good friend Prof. Cui as well when I conclude that our cooperation has been quite fruitful, not only for our own career, but also for our students, not only for science, but also for practical dental and medical applications, and last but not least, for both of our countries.

# 2.3 A Life of Engineering Innovation Founded on Lessons from Nature

Myron Spector

Department of Orthopedics, Brigham and Women's Hospital,
Harvard Medical School, Boston, MA
Tissue Engineering, VA Boston Healthcare System, Boston, MA

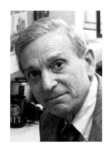

Myron Spector，美国哈佛大学教授，哈佛大学医学院生物材料研究室主任，麻省理工学院材料科学与工程系高级讲师。2003 年美国生物材料学会主席。美国 FDA 骨科器械专家组组长（1998—2014 年）。主要研究领域为生物材料、组织工程与再生医学材料。

Knowledge and ideas come to those attentive to lessons that nature has to teach. That pursuit is embodied in "biomimetics". Fu-Zhai Cui has been one of the most successful practitioners of the biomimetic engineering approach, and an excellent role model for young scientists.

The premier product that Prof. Cui engineered, Bongold TM Bone Graft Replacement, is a novel and effective bone graft substitute material, which is used for the treatment of several clinical problems including spine fusion. The product, approved several years ago by the CFDA, is sold throughout China and in Vietnam, and has recently been approved by the US FDA for sale in the US. The porous material is a composite of nano-apatite and collagen fabricated by a novel method that allows for the coordinated self-assembly of the material[1,2]. Professor Cui conceived of the bone graft product, developed the novel method of fabrication, and was the principal investigator of laboratory and animal pre-clinical investigations[1-8], and a collaborator in the human trials. Prof. Cui's work was highlighted in Research Notes of *Nature*

*Materials* 2003, which commented that: "These results should improve the under-standing of collagen-mediated mineralization in other calcified tissues, and point the way to new functional materials for biomimetic engineering."

Prof. Cui's scholarly work that formed the foundation of his approach to developing the nano-apatite/collagen/PLA composite included fundamental studies of the structure and properties of bone[9,10], fracture callus[11-13], and bones of mutant Zebrafish[14-16], studies based on lessons from nature. The latter work was particularly innovative as it allowed for the determination of the structure-properties relationships for genetically altered bone.

I have known Prof. Cui for 20 years and have collaborated with him on several projects[17-19]. He served as a Visiting Scholar (in residence) at the Massachusetts Institute of Technology for 3 months in 1997. A few years later, Prof. Cui and I created a graduate level course that we co-taught as a joint endeavor of Harvard–MIT and Tsinghua: "HST535 Principles and Practice of Tissue Engineering". For 3 years, the subject was taught in English via video conference in the Fall term (8 : 00– 9 : 30 AM Boston time). This demonstrated Prof. Cui's commitment to biomaterials education as well as research, and his facility for working in the English language.

In underscoring how Prof. Cui utilized basic knowledge in science to accomplish a significant goal in the biomaterials area, it is important to note the following. During the period that Prof. Cui was researching and developing his bone graft substitute material, there was a substantial amount of effort worldwide directed toward this same goal. However, Prof. Cui's development was not a "me-too" product. His scientific work, informed by his many prior studies of the structure-properties relationships of osseous tissues, led him to develop a new method of coordinated self-assembly of a nano-apatite/collagen composite, reflecting to some extent the process by which bone itself mineralizes. While others had demonstrated self-assembly phenomena using peptides and other biomolecules, Prof. Cui was the first to implement the coordinated self-assembly of a material using a 2-component system, nano-apatite and collagen. This discovery allowed for the development of a scaffold for bone regeneration with properties that could not otherwise have been achieved.

It is also important to highlight the fact that Prof. Cui has been responsible for important biomaterials research focused on the treatment of diverse medical problems. He pioneered studies to employ biomaterials for treating brain lesions, and could be credited with the creation of an entirely new field, brain tissue engineering. He completed animal (rat) studies that demonstrated that biomaterial scaffolds can be used as delivery vehicles for antagonists (viz., antibodies) of molecules that inhibit nerve regeneration ( viz. , Nogo) . These novel biomaterials, when implanted into lesions in the rat brain, could ameliorate behavioral deficits, and facilitate the processes that underlie positive reparative responses. His studies inspired our own in this area.

When the prestigious publisher, the Institute of Physics in the United Kingdom, decided to launch a biomaterials journal, they turned to Prof. Cui to be Editor-in-Chief. In his unselfish way, Prof. Cui asked me and his colleague, In-Seop Lee from Seoul, Korea, to join him as co-Editors-in-Chief. Due to other demands on his time, Professor Cui stepped down from editorship position in 2010. The journal that he started continues to thrive, with a current Impact Factor of 3. 697.

In many ways Fu-Zhai remains, even at 70, a student himself. He continues to be enthusiastic in his seeking new knowledge and excited by the prospect of developing innovative medical devices. In this, and in many other ways, he continues to serve as an inspiration to young scientists, and to old colleagues like me.

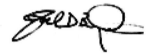

# References

[1]    Liao S S, Cui F Z. In vitro and in vivo degradation of mineralized collagen-based composite scaffold: Nanohydroxyapatite/collagen/poly ( L-lactide) [J]. *Tissue Engineering*, 2004, 10 (1-2): 73-80.

[2]    Liao S S, Cui F Z, Zhang W, et al. Hierarchically biomimetic bone scaffold materials: Nano-HA/collagen/PLA composite [J]. *Journal of Biomedical Materials Research Part B : Applied Biomaterials*, 2004, 69B (2): 158-165.

[3]    Zhang S M, Cui F Z, Liao S S, et al. Synthesis and biocompatibility of porous nano-hydroxyapatite/collagen/alginate composite [J]. *Journal of Materials Science*, 2003, 14 (7): 641-645.

[4]    Sun T S, Guan K, Shi S S, et al. Effect of nano-hydroxyapatite/collagen composite and bone morphogenetic protein-2 on lumbar intertransverse fusion in rabbits [J]. *Chinese Journal of Traumatology*, 2004, 7 (1): 18-24.

[5]    Liao S S, Guan K, Cui F Z, et al. Lumbar spinal fusion with a mineralized collagen matrix and rhBMP-2 in a rabbit model [J]. *Spine*, 2003, 28 (17): 1954-1960.

[6]    Du C, Cui F Z, Zhang W, et al. Formation of calcium phosphate/collagen composites through mineralization of collagen matrix [J]. *Journal of Biomedical Materials Research*,

2000, 50 (4): 518-527.

[ 7 ]  Du C, Cui F Z, Zhu X D, et al. Three-dimensional nano-HAp/collagen matrix loading with osteogenic cells in organ culture [J]. *Journal of Biomedical Materials Research*, 1999, 44 (4): 407-415.

[ 8 ]  Du C, Cui F Z, Feng Q L, et al. Tissue response to nano-hydroxyapatite/collagen composite implants in marrow cavity [J]. *Journal of Biomedical Materials Research*, 1998, 42 (4): 540-548.

[ 9 ]  Su X, Sun K, Cui F Z, et al. Organization of apatite crystals in human woven bone [J]. *Bone*, 2003, 32 (2): 150-162.

[ 10 ]  Su X W, Feng Q L, Cui F Z, et al. Microstructure and micromechanical properties of the middiaphyses of human fetal femurs [J]. *Connective Tissue Research*, 1997, 36 (3): 271-286.

[ 11 ]  Wen H B, Cui F Z, Zhu X D. Microstructural features of non-union of human humeral shaft fracture [J]. *Journal of Structural Biology*, 1997, 119 (3): 239-246.

[ 12 ]  Cui F Z, Wen H B, Su X W, et al. Microstructures of external periosteal callus of repaired femoral fracture in children [J]. *Journal of Structural Biology*, 1996, 117 (3): 204-208.

[ 13 ]  Wen H B, Cui F Z, Feng Q L, et al. Microstructural investigation of the early external callus after diaphyseal fractures of human long bone [J]. *Journal of Structural Biology*, 1995, 114 (2): 115-122.

[ 14 ]  Wang X M, Cui F Z, Ge J, et al. Hierarchical structural comparisons of bones from wild-type and liliput (dtc232) gene-mutated zebrafish [J]. *Journal of Structural Biology*, 2004, 145 (3): 236-245.

[ 15 ]  Wang X M, Cui F Z, Ge J, et al. Variation of nanomechanical properties of bone by gene mutation in the zebrafish [J]. *Biomaterials*, 2002, 23 (23): 4557-4563.

[ 16 ]  Zhang Y, Cui F Z, Wang X M, et al. Mechanical properties of skeletal bone in gene-mutated stopsel (dtl28d) and wild-type zebrafish (Danio rerio) measured by atomic force microscopy-based nanoindentation [J]. *Bone*, 2002, 30 (4): 541-546.

[ 17 ]  Comut A A, Weber H P, Shortkroff S, et al. Connective tissue orientation around dental implants in a canine model [J]. *Clinical Oral Implants Research*, 2001, 12 (5): 433-440.

[ 18 ]  Ma J, Tian W M, Hou S P, et al. An experimental test of stroke recovery by implanting a hyaluronic acid hydrogel carrying a Nogo receptor antibody in a rat model [J]. *Biomedical Materials*, 2007, 2 (4): 233-240.

[ 19 ]  Tian W M, Hou S P, Ma J, et al. Hyaluronic acid-poly-D-lysine-based three-dimensional hydrogel for traumatic brain injury [J]. *Tissue Engineering*, 2005, 11 (3-4): 513-525.

# 2.4　Friendship with Prof. Fu-Zhai Cui

In-Seop Lee

Yonsei University, Seoul, South Korea

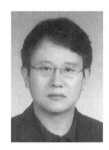
In-Seop Lee，1996 年获美国辛辛那提大学博士学位。生物陶瓷和再生医学材料专家，韩国延世大学生物材料教授。国际刊物 *Biomedical Materials* 主编（2010—），曾任 8 届中韩生物材料研讨会韩方主席（2007—2014 年）。在韩国培养、联合培养 10 名以上中国研究生。

It's my great pleasure and honor to contribute an article to the book titled "How to make creativities in biomaterials" for celebrating Prof. Cui's 70th birthday. As many his intimate colleagues and former students will describe his professional excellence such as his leadership in the field of biomaterials, passion, insight, and endeavor to both students and research, I'd like to mention some of my personal experiences and relationships with him to share how great and warm heart person he is.

I have known Prof. Cui since the first China–Korea Symposium on Ion Beam Modification of Materials held at Tsinghua University in 1993 (Photo 2.1) at which we both served as a general secretary. Although the diplomatic relationship between Korea and China was established in 1992, visiting China required not only visa but also special permission from our government. But such complication processes could not stop us to communicate and collaborate. We visited each lab regularly and advised students (Photo 2.2, B-H Zhao who became a professor of China Medical University in Shenyang, China). We also reported and published our cooperative results to the high ranked scientific journals and the international conferences (Photo 2.3, 2007 Asian-European International Conference on Plasma Surface Engineering held in Nagasaki, Japan and Photo 2.4, 2007 Annual Meeting of Society for Biomaterials held in Chicago, USA). In 2003, we established China-Korea Symposium on Biomaterials and Nano-Bio Technology with financial support from both countries (the 2011 symposium held in Sanya, China), and it still holds annually.

In 2005, He, I and Prof. M. Spector discussed to launch the new scientific journal entitled "*Biomedical Materials*" (Photo 2.5, Shanghai, China) and published the first issue in 2006. I sincerely admire his professional achievements and also congratulate his 70th birthday. Prof. Cui is my best colleague and friend although we are different in age and nationality.

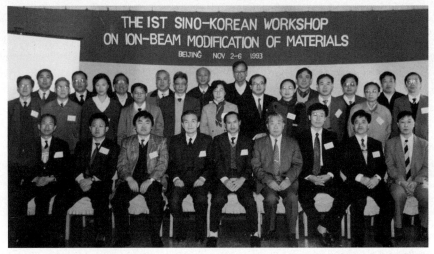

Photo 2.1　1993 年在清华大学召开的中韩会议，前排左 4 是清华大学杨家庆常务副校长

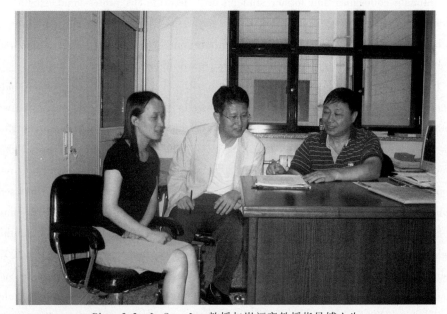

Photo 2.2　In-Seop Lee 教授与崔福斋教授指导博士生

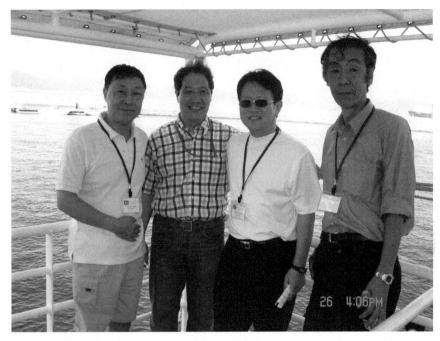

Photo 2.3　2007 年 AEPSE 会议期间在韩国汉江上 In-Seop Lee 教授、Takya 教授、
崔福斋教授等合影

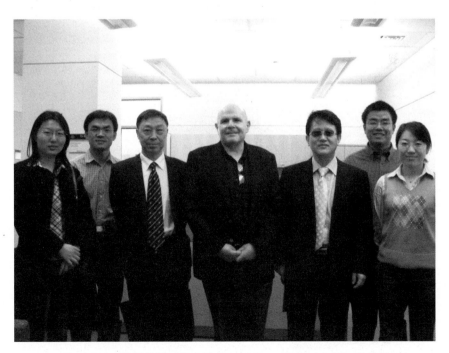

Photo 2.4　访问美国西北大学 Samuel Stupp 教授（中间）办公室

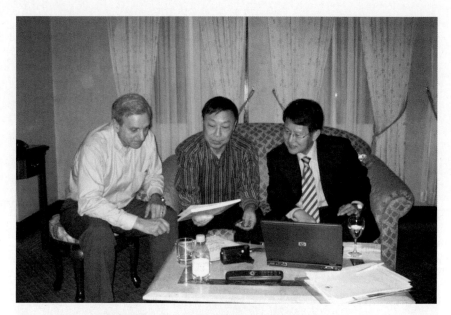

Photo 2.5 *Biomedical Materials* 的三位主编讨论

# 2.5 Pioneer to Drive a New Frontier of Biomaterials Science

Fumio Watari

Graduate School of Dental Medicine, Hokkaido University,
Sapporo, Japan

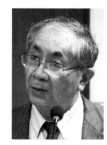

Fumio Watari，日本北海道大学生物材料教授。本科、硕士以及博士均毕业于日本东京大学，之后到欧洲和美国工作 6 年，从 1993 年起任北海道大学教授。主要从事微米/纳米颗粒的毒理学和生物医学应用、碳纳米管及其衍生物的生物医学应用等领域的研究。

## 1. Nano, Bio, Regenerative

Materials act on biological body with their chemical properties, mostly through the form of ions or small molecules. The effects are originated from materials themselves and non-biological, which works irrespective of the conditions whether biological body exists or not. When materials become nano in size, they start to have physically interactive nature with biological body at the level of cells and tissue, in addition to the chemical effects. The biointeraction at the cellular or subcellular level makes arise the biological process to lead to inflammation or tissue regeneration, depending on the situated circumstances inside biological body. Thus the biointeractive nature induces the nano specific functions through biological process, which are not originally possessed in materials and different from non-biological effect. This effect appears only under the conditions of both existence of nanomaterials and biological body.

For the long time, the role of materials on medicine has been limited. Materials have been used mostly for the therapy of hard tissue, bone and teeth, in the field of orthopedics and dentistry such as implant which remains as foreign object in a bioadaptive manner inside body. However, most of the fields of medicine except orthopae-dics treat soft tissue and use pharmacological agents as the main curing means to as-sist self-recovery force or body defense system. By inducing nano, materials start to have the biologically interactive potential and acquire the function to work from bioin-ert, biosympathetic, biopositive to bioactive, biointeractive and bioreactive nature[1].

The potentiality of bioactive function possessed by nanomaterials can propose to be applicable for tissue regeneration. The success or not of tissue or organ regeneration stands on the fundamentals of the choice of biomaterials, in addition to those of stem cells and differentiating agents. At this stage thus the biointeraction potential of mate-rials can propose the contribution different from drugs to medicine, which opens the new horizon of regenerative medicine or cancer therapy.

Prof. Cui had the insights for the future possibility of nano functions in biomateri-als, initiated and driven investigations forward, invented biomimetic structure, and developed regenerative materials which are now further on the way to regenerative medicine.

One of the typical examples is the nano-apatite collagen composites strengthened with bioresorptive polymer, which gives the regenerative nature of bone and bone substitute functions. Conventionally apatite or titanium has so far been used as foreign object adaptive to body but they are not substitutable to natural bone. This nano-in-ducing regenerative model is now advancing to the field of soft tissue for the regenera-tion of neuron, recovery of brain damage or other organs.

Prof. Cui has thus pioneered the field of nano effect on biomaterials, developed nano biomaterials, regenerative materials to nano biomedicine, regenerative medi-cine, and is now still promoting the progress.

## 2. Working attitude for action and enterprise

Thus Prof. Cui has made academic accomplishments in the field of biomaterials, and opened the new world in biomaterial science and nanomedicine. His activity is not only limited in the basic academism. He works very actively to promote the new field with many scientists in the international level. He planned the project, hosted many international congresses, and set up the plural new international scientific journals. He has done the investigation, directed experiments, developed the regenerative nanomaterials to clinical application with practice, patents, and commercial medical devices. He educated many young students grown to excellent researchers, which is his another great accomplishments to influence on the field of science in the world.

The details of these accomplishments will be more suitably described by other peo-ple. Here I would like to describe more his working style and personality as researcher of science with which I have acquainted during the contact up to now and are impressed.

Prof. Cui's working style is simple, quick and decisive. He grasps the cores of problems, gets into the heart of essence and necessities, proposes the idea and plans with significance, and acts into practice vital for realization. His mind is bright, open, generous, friendly, direct without unnecessary politeness. His accomplishments are great but he is very modest and polite to the other people with accomplishments.

His talent, character, activities are as above and it would be enough to explain. If it is still insufficient, we may explain in other way as follows: he is not the person who has become great by tactics, graciousness or sociability. He proposes the original ideas, show and share the chances with other people, drives for further enterprise and future targets, and these result in the present status.

When I try to explain, Prof. Cui's personality, talent, working style, characters, and driving force to develop the new scientific region recalls me of the words by Tullius Cicero, ancient Roman philosopher and orator, on Caesar. Julius Caesar is, of course, famous in history, but he is also well-known with his brief, simple and vivid usage of words such as "Veni, vidi, vici" (came, saw, won). Cicero expressed the remark on Caesar's description "Commentary on the Gallic War", one of the most popular classics and often used as textbook for the beginners of Latin literature, as follows:

" ⋯ splendid! ⋯ It is bare, straight and handsome, stripped of rhetorical ornament like an athlete off away his clothes. ⋯ Nothing is more sweet, attractive than pure and clear brevity. ⋯ "

Prof. Cui's work, activity, speed and spirit impresses me that such adjectives are proper to express them.

## 3. Prof. Cui's world

I first met Prof. Cui in 2001 when China-Japan Seminar on Functionally Graded Materials (FGM) was held in Tsinghua University. He invited me to visit his laboratory. I was impressed with the activity of his laboratory and at the same time with many excellent students.

In the aspect of international standard, Tsinghua University is the one that the most excellent students gather with the talent potential to work actively in all over the world.

Then I had the chance to invite Prof. Cui in 2002 and another for 5th Asian Bio-Ceramics Symposium (ABC2005) with his young pupils. One of them is Prof. Xiang-Dong Kong who works now in Zhejiang sci-tech University. After time is passed, I have forgotten completely those things. But Prof. Cui occasionally and repetitively talked about that. In other time Prof. Kong also reminded me of that. Then some old memory comes out to me. I found a few photos, although there should be more somewhere. Photo 2.6 is in front of Edo (old name of Tokyo) period heritage Red Gate (17th century) of Tokyo University. Photo 2.7 is at Edo period-like cultural snack bar. They have many lanterns on the roof with the name of contributors to snack which are not seen in this photo.

I was happy to host the excellent young researchers from his laboratory, Prof. Su-San Liao (now in National University of Singapore) and Prof. Xiao-Ming Li (Beihang University), as postdoctors for two years with JSPS (Japanese Society for Promotion of Science) Postdoctoral Fellowship in our laboratory. They had researches with unique ideas and developed to publish many accomplishments. For international symposium, we could have the attendance from Prof. Cui's laboratory or biomaterial group. In Photo 2.8 at ABC2005, Prof. Cui is in the center and Prof. Kong a little left in the middle row.

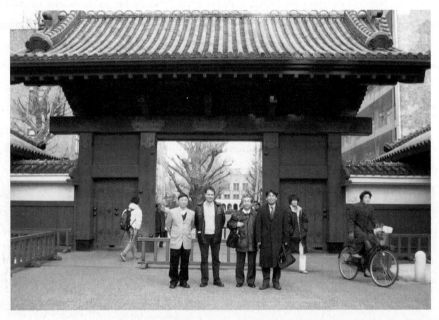

Photo 2.6　崔福斋在北海道大学做访问学者

I have visited China several times, which is much more than other countries and more than I expected before. That is because I got to know Prof. Cui, attended his organizing international congresses, got acquainted with his young researchers and students, then they have become professors and independent researchers in many

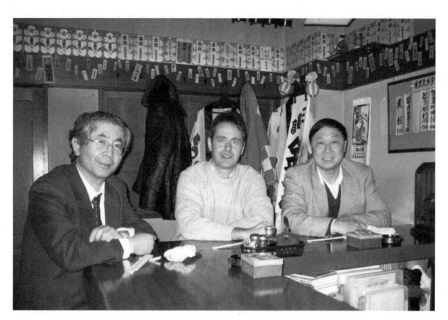

Photo 2.7　在 Watari 教授办公室

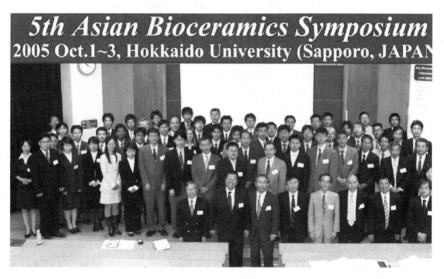

Photo 2.8　在日本札幌北海道大学召开的国际会议

highly reputed universities in China, now they themselves organize the international symposium and I attend also these or have invitation. China is wide, and I had chances to visit various area. In addition to Prof. Qing-Ling Feng, Prof. Cai, Prof. Wang and Prof. Li in Beijing, I visited Prof. Kong in Hangzhou, Prof. Qiang Lu and Dr. Xi Liu (now in Yale University, USA) at Soochow University in Suzhou, and Prof. Xiao-Jie Lian (Taiyuan University of Technology) in Taiyuan and others, also with the advice of Prof. Li who invited me plural times. If I had not been acquainted with Prof. Cui, my visit to China would have been much more rare.

It is somewhat like the Sun Wukong (Monkey in the tale of Journey to the West of the Monk Xuanzang at the time of Tang dynasty) who makes a violate activity to demonstrate his mighty power but after a while he notices that it is the play done just on the hand palm of Buddha. I am just like a dancer on Prof. Cui's palm.

Prof. Cui has brought up many excellent students. Every time to visit his laboratory or attend international symposium, I saw they work hard brightly and vividly under the directorship of Prof. Cui. Now they are grown up to be at the important position in the renowned universities, institutes or companies all over the world. The impression that I had got from them is that they are not only excellent, active, positive, but also friendly, sincere, reliable and bright.

I enjoy the merit on the heaven of Prof. Cui's world. At the same time the abundance of excellent members flourishing from Prof. Cui's school is one of the most impressive, admirable and also enviable accomplishments.

## 4. Great spirits that I have met in my life

I was graduated originally as metallurgist, then became electron microscopist, covered as material scientist, finally work as dental and biomaterial scientist. During these days, I have contacted great spirits. Prof. S. Amelinckx (Belgian Atomic Institute and University of Antwerp (RUCA), Belgium) was well-known for the achievements in the field of application of electron microscopy for crystallography and the analysis of phase and lattice defects of materials and minerals. He wrote one paper during one air flight every time he got on like a hobby, while he worked as general director in the atomic institute. Prof. J. M. Cowley (Arizona State University, USA) established the atomic image high resolution electron microscopy, together with Prof. Sumio Iijima who is now more known as the discoverer of carbon nanotubes. Then I met Prof. Cui in the field of biomaterials.

Prof. Cui's activity and accomplishments override the border of nations. Originality of research, editors including newly founded journals, research grants, numbers and excellence of his school pupils, organization of international congresses, academic positions, international acquaintances, medical applications, patents, venture companies, influence on international academic societies—When I consider over these, I wonder who can surpass him. I have come into the conclusion such that it is difficult to surpass him in any aspects.

## 5. Other aspects

Along with the strong will for active working, Prof. Cui is very strong with alcohols and many of his excellent disciples are also similarly strong and love drinks. He provides such occasions to have a pleasant time together with his pupils and guests from foreign countries, and there are many things to talk about life, however for this subject I should yield the opportunity to someone else.

## 6. Congratulations and wish for the future

Prof. Cui has attained seventy years old. The accomplishments that he has done up to now is already great enough, however, it seems to me that it is not all that he can do or he should do in his life. What he should do in his life has not been attained yet. Society will need his activity, opinion, proposals and directorship.

Herewith I congratulate Prof. Cui's 70th year anniversary and at the same time wish he will drive the horizon of the new scientific world further for the future!

# Reference

[1]    Watari F, Takashi N, Yokoyama A, et al. Material nanosizing effect on living organisms: Non-specific, biointeractive, physical size effects [J]. *J. Roy. Soc. Interface*, 2009, 6: S371-S388.

# 2.6　生物材料与人生

汪日志

英属哥伦比亚大学材料工程系，加拿大

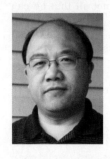

汪日志，加拿大英属哥伦比亚大学材料工程系教授，生物医学工程系和骨科系教授。1983 年，于浙江大学获得学士学位；1993 年，于哈尔滨工业大学材料科学与工程系获得博士学位；1993—1995 年，在清华大学从事博士后研究。2002—2012 年，担任加拿大生物材料协会主席；2012—2013 年，担任加拿大生物材料学会主席。目前主要从事关节修复及替代相关材料的研究。

　　1993 年博士答辩后，坐了两天两夜的车从哈尔滨回到浙江老家。才住了一天，就接到崔老师从北京打来的电话，要我在放暑假前去清华报到。第二天，我赶紧乘汽车又转火车赶去北京。崔老师骑着自行车载着我一个办公室又一个办公室地办手续。就这样，我在 1993 年的夏天第一次见到崔老师并开始了在清华的博士后研究。

　　我先后在国内外 8 个大学学习、工作过，每个学校的校风都不一样。清华大学的学术风气很浓，工字厅里办事效率也很高。感觉有点像我后来工作过的普林斯顿大学，带点历史，带点骄傲。我理解的校风不仅包括实验室与教室里的笔记与辩论，更体现在大街上的人流交错。与北美的大学相比，清华大学虽然少了那些能随时随意坐下聊天的咖啡厅，却多了规模巨大的餐厅与赏心悦目的小桥流水。当年，买上三食堂的可口美食，坐在荷塘小亭里与同仁谈古论今的情景，至今记忆犹新。记忆中还有清华大学那潮水一样的自行车流，潮水一样地去教室、去新东方，又潮水一样地回宿舍。清华园的自行车总是那么整齐地排着，与邻居北京大学的截然不同。这也许是工科生的严谨吧。

　　我就是在这样一个环境里开始我的博士后研究的。当时，李恒德教授与崔福斋教授这两位合作导师的科研侧重有所不同。李先生个人对材料仿生比较感兴趣，而崔老师更加侧重生物医用材料。80 年代末、90 年代初，世界各国材料界都在设法从传统的冶金领域拓展，开辟新的方向。生物仿生及生物医用材料正是在这一背景下兴起的。以美国材料研究协会年会为代表的国际会议每年都有专题分会讨论这一方向，参加的人数也不断增加。现在大部分材料系都设有这方面的研究组，生物医用材料产业也已形成相当规模。所以当时李先生与崔老师在确定研究方向时还是很有远见的。

经过短暂论证后，我提出博士后研究从贝壳的结构、力学与仿生着手。贝壳珍珠层是材料仿生领域最熟知的天然生物材料。虽然其成分中的95%以上是方解石，珍珠层却拥有了普通陶瓷材料并不具有的高韧性。它的强韧性现象在90年代初由当时西雅图华盛顿大学的Aksay教授在几次材料研究协会年会冬季会议上引入美国材料界，引起广泛关注。当时，美国正在全力解决结构陶瓷的脆性问题，对贝壳珍珠层等天然生物材料韧性的研究可以给组织与结构设计带来灵感。我当时对这一全新的仿生概念很感兴趣。从课题可行性而言，贝壳虽然是天然生物材料，但研究所使用的基本方法和实验手段与传统材料研究大致相同，起步相对容易。研究计划得到了李、崔两位导师的支持。当时，组里前期已有人做了一些晶体取向与成分分析工作，于是我决定从显微结构与力学行为关系着手。后来几个月实验的辛苦以及熬夜写论文在此略过。实验结果即使在现在看来都很有意思。文章写好后，崔老师逐行逐字改过，研究报告顺利发表[1,2]。这阶段在贝壳上的研究与其说是对清华大学研究组的贡献，倒不如说是开启了我今后几十年的一个重要研究方向。五六年后，有机会在普林斯顿大学与Aksay教授、Evans教授以及锁志刚教授合作，重启这一课题，对贝壳珍珠层的一些特性有了全新的认识[3,4]，这是后话。

崔老师对生物医用材料及生物矿化仍是情有独钟。当时，研究组在这个方向的情形是，除了钱、人，什么都没有。钱是李先生、崔老师争取来的。人是清华大学吸引来的。当时，生物材料方向有直博的温海波，读硕士的卢红波（马春雷老师的学生），后来加入了杜昶、苏晓维。做科研的人都知道，经费与学生是决定因素。尽管如此，万事开头难。崔老师带我们去清华大学生物系，实验上得到了那里老师们的大力协助。北京大学生物系实验室也对我们热情开放。崔老师还热情邀请了中日友好医院骨科的朱晓东医生。朱医生非常敬业，敢于动手。由于与他的合作，我也因此有机会了解到临床上遇到的材料问题。当时的情形是，我在清华大学制备材料，朱医生在医院做动物实验。虽然忘了结果如何，但当时的合作让我看到了生物材料研究中与临床医生合作的必要性。多年以后，当我在加拿大英属哥伦比亚大学确立研究组的研究策略时，与骨科大夫的合作自然地成了首选。

记得有一次与崔老师一起从工物馆骑车出来，崔老师说他开始对胶原感兴趣。当时，我在看生物化学方面的书，也在研究骨头力学和矿化，对胶原在书面上有些了解，但对怎么在实验室里利用胶原做生物材料还是一窍不通。当时，我大胆地做了一件事：花天价从 Sigma 公司买来 I 型可溶胶原。忘记了崔老师在报账签字时是否皱过眉头，反正骨科用生物材料制备就这么开始了。我根据骨头的基本成分，结合所学到的矿化机理，制备了胶原/羟基磷灰石复合材料。论文以 Letter 形式发表[5]。这一工作在现在看来非常简单，但从当时的课题发展来说应该是重要的一步。我本人也从研究中积累了经验，为以后的生物材料研究打下了基础。

回顾清华两年以及后来多年的研究经历，我觉得一个多学科交叉的研究课题对研究者既是机会又是挑战。即使有各学科专家的合作，研究者只有敢于跨越学科界限，才能找到共同语言，充分利用相关学科的优势。

团队文化在科学研究中不仅影响当时的科研进展，更影响研究人员今后的发展道路。崔老师在团队建设上做了不少努力。黄师母曾说过，崔老师是个好人。我的理解是，崔老师说话直接，做事实在。由此引申开来，当时，研究组老师有李先生、崔老师、马春雷老师，后来又加入了冯庆玲老师。团队日常的合作与交流应该是崔老师在主导的。当时，组里的学术活动就是按现在的标准去衡量也算是相当活跃和国际化的。我们与北京大学医学部的王嶶教授研究组有不定期的学术交流；崔老师还专门带我们去北京大学人民医院等地方听学术报告。国际交流上，崔老师就已跟哈佛大学开始神经修复方面的合作探索。中间我还去澳大利亚 Perth 参加了一次国际会议，认识了澳大利亚生物矿化领域领军人 John Webb 教授。Steve Weiner 教授是国际生物矿化方面的权威，他一直关注清华大学生物材料的发展。1995 年，他借来北京周口店考古的机会到清华大学做过一场很有意思的报告。我知道后来还来过多次。Weiner 教授也是我离开清华大学之后从事博士后研究的合作导师。当时，组里的一次大练兵是崔老师 1994 年组织的中韩材料表面改性双边会议。参加者包括崔老师以后几十年一直合作的 In-Seop Lee 教授。组里学生们承担的任务主要是发信、引路这些琐碎工作。但我在这次会议中体会到的那种国际化气氛是非常强烈的。

记忆中，组里师生之间的关系是非常融洽的。崔老师不惜掏腰包带我们一起去卡拉 OK，去中关村必胜客尝鲜，去吃韩国烧烤……在外国人眼中，中国人喜欢吃，近年来，随着交流多了，也重新认识了这种文化。老祖宗们很早就知道，人在放开胃口时，也打开了心扉，交流也因此变得容易了。交流沟通在生意场重要，在科研界也必不可少，只是各国流行的方法各有不同。

游历各国多年深切体会到，科学研究表面上看来是人对自然界的探索，但实际上是人与人的交流，是人对社会的探索。发表的文章会随着科研的发展被渐渐淡忘，但遇到过的人和经过的事会深深地烙在记忆中，变得越来越珍贵。当 20 年后我在广州珠江边再次碰到 In-Seop Lee 教授时，当同样 20 年后在加拿大的 Saskatoon 与中日友好医院的朱医生重逢时，我深切地体会到这一点。

# 参考文献

[1]    Wang R Z, Wen H B, Cui F Z, et al. Observations on the damage morphologies of nacre during deformation and fracture [J]. *Journal of Materials Science*, 1995, 30: 2299-2304.

[2]    Wang R Z, Cui F Z, Feng Q L, et al. Development of biomimetic designed alumina/fiber reinforced epoxy laminated composite [J]. *Journal of Materials Research*, 1996, 10: 95-100.

[3]    Wang R Z, Suo Z, Evans A G, et al. Deformation mechanisms in nacre [J]. *Journal of Materials Research*, 2001, 16: 2485-2493.

[4]    Evans A G, Suo Z, Wang R Z, et al. A model for the resilient mechanical behavior of nacre [J]. *Journal of Materials Research*, 2001, 16: 2475-2484.

[5]    Wang R Z, Cui F Z, Lu H B, et al. Synthesis of nanophase hydroxyapatite/ collagen composite [J]. *Journal of Materials Science Letters*, 1995, 14: 490-492.

# 2.7 献给崔福斋教授 70 岁生日

唐睿康

浙江大学，杭州

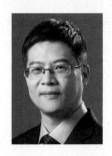

唐睿康，浙江大学化学系教授，教育部"长江学者奖励计划"特聘教授，浙江省特聘专家。浙江大学生物物质与信息调控研究中心主任，浙江大学求是高等研究院成员。中国化学会理事，杭州市青年科技工作者协会会长，浙江大学青年教授联谊会副会长。中国青年科技奖获得者。主要从事生物矿化研究。

崔老师与中国生物矿化研究的起步和发展紧密联系在一起，他不仅是生物矿化领域的领军人物，也是我在这个研究方向上的重要领路人之一。20 世纪90 年代初，我在南京大学求学期间第一次接触到生物矿化。早期生物矿化研究的一个重要方向就是对生物材料结构的观测，那时候人们刚认识到生物矿化材料中的分级结构及其重要性，其中唯一可以找到的来自中国的原创性研究就是崔老师基于象牙的观测提出了牙的分级结构。这一成果随着生物矿化的发展被大量引用，为生物矿化材料的分级构筑这一核心概念的发展做出了重要的贡献。我还记得，导师郁子厚教授在向我传授生物矿化知识时就专门介绍了崔老师的工作。尽管那时我还不认识崔老师，但他的名字和成果已经带领着我进入了生物矿化这片天地。

崔老师的研究思路开阔，具有很好的研究前瞻性。他很早就胶原-磷酸钙体系开展研究，通过大量细致的观测证实了在生物矿化的早期阶段，胶原能够调制纳米晶羟基磷灰石在其表面的取向沉积，进而组装为矿化胶原纤维簇，证实了长期以来的猜想。该成果发表后得到了学术界的广泛好评，其中 *Nature Materials* 的评价是"……给出支持矿化胶原理论的第一个直接实验证据……"目前，胶原矿化已经发展成为生物矿化中最重要的一个体系，而崔老师在这一方面的成就是先驱性的，并奠定了很好的基础，这使他的学生在后续的发展中能够在这一领域做出更大的突破，例如，杜昶博士关于蛋白矿化及组装的工作

发表在 *Science* 上。

崔老师还特别重视学科交叉，他给我留下的另一个深刻印象就是 2002 年在高登研究会议上关于斑马鱼成骨的研究报告。在这个研究中，他将生物基因技术引入生物矿化中，从而可以从生物角度调控骨形成过程。这个报告对我后来的发展有很大启示和影响，例如，目前我的研究特别重视材料和生物的相互结合，从不同学科角度研究生物矿化，但此前往往局限在物理和化学之中。

崔老师对我的重要影响还有"要做有用的研究"，对此他不仅给我很多的教导，更是用他自己的实际行动来引导我。崔老师的研究工作特点是将机制理论和实际应用通过生物矿化进行了完美结合。他研究中的科学问题来自自然实际，所取得的成果也能指导实际应用。例如，他将胶原矿化机制探索和骨修复材料的开发有机地联系在一起，通过机制探索设计出可以促进骨修复的新型纳米晶磷酸钙材料，特别值得一提的是，在临床应用中也得到了成功的验证，是生物材料"研究—开发—临床"的范例。崔老师不仅是一位科学家，而且是一位创业家，成功地把实验室的研究成果转化为产品推向了市场，为社会的发展做出了切实的贡献，得到病人和医生的认可应该是这项研究的最高荣誉。我们不仅为崔老师所取得的成就感到骄傲，更为他的境界和勇气感到敬佩。虽然在科研和产业的结合上，我还没有崔老师这样的魄力和能力，但他给我们树立了一个很好的榜样，这也促使我在科研中特别注意"有用性"这个大方向的把握。我会要求学生简练准确地说出他们所开展每一项研究的"有用性"，而正是这个"有用性"激发学生积极主动开展基础的科研工作。

崔老师对生物矿化研究的贡献还有很多体现在科研工作之外。他的心胸宽广，工作并不局限在实验室，还投入了大量额外的精力用以推动学术交流，创办并主办了各类生物矿化相关会议（例如亚洲生物矿化会议及国际生物矿化会议），还主持了一系列高水平学术期刊的建设，为广大研究者提供成果和信息的交流平台。他的科研责任感不仅得到了国际同行的高度好评，也使他成为国际生物矿化领域的代表人物。这些努力也很好地推动了国内生物矿化研究的发展，使我们都成为直接的受益者。崔老师所主编的《生物矿化》一书已经成为这个领域的经典之作，在为研究者提供系统的参考指导的同时，还启蒙了更多青年人投身到生物矿化的事业中。还需要一提的是，他是我们国家自然科学基金委员会第一个生物矿化跨学科重点项目的负责人之一，也是我们领域第一个荣获国家自然科学奖二等奖的学者，这很好地体现了崔老师对生物矿化研究所做出的杰出贡献。

虽然我并不是崔老师名义上的学生，但在我的心里，崔老师就是我的导师。在我的科研道路上，到处都可以看到崔老师对我的感召和影响。特别是我回国工作后，崔老师在各个方面给了我很多的指导、帮助和鼓励，使我能够很好地适应新的环境并开辟新的研究天地。我也特地借此机会向崔老师表示衷心的感谢！祝崔老师 70 周岁生日快乐！更重要的是，我们要向崔老师学习，学习他的科学精神，踏踏实实地将研究工作做好、做透，在科学创新中坚持理论联系应用，使生物矿化研究领域更好、更快地发展壮大。

# 2.8  科研道路的选择：兴趣与坚持

## 孙晓丹

清华大学材料学院，北京

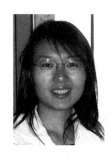

孙晓丹，清华大学材料学院副研究员。1993 年，于清华大学攻读学士学位；1998 年，免试攻读博士学位；2004 年初留校任教。一直从事纳米材料的仿生制备与应用研究，在美国哈佛大学留学期间（2006 年 8 月—2007 年 8 月），开始全面转入生物医用材料的研究工作。

　　1993 年，我从河北省邯郸市第一中学考入清华大学材料科学与工程系，攻读学士学位。高中时自己就很喜欢生物，但那年清华大学生物系在邯郸不招生，也便作罢。后来听说在材料科学与工程系有个生物材料研究组，兴趣便又被激发出来，从本科开始到硕博连读，连续六七年间都在这个组内学习。崔老师常爱跟别人介绍说我是他的"小师妹"，这个辈分源于我们两人共同的博士导师——中国材料届的泰斗李恒德院士。崔老师是李先生的第一位博士生，而我是李先生的最后一位直博生。

　　李先生在我做博士课题选择时很关注"自组装"这个过程仿生的概念，因此，我和另一位博士生王毓德（现云南大学教授）的课题就是利用自组装方法制备纳米/介孔结构的过渡金属氧化物。当时，这个方向在国际上是很热门的一个研究领域，而我们对多种金属氧化物进行了比较系统的研究工作，相关工作获得了云南省科学技术奖——云南省自然科学奖二等奖，其中一篇文章 *Preparation of nanocrystalline metal oxide powders with the surfactant-mediated method* 至今已被引用 106 次。但当时我制备的那些材料并不是用于生物医学领域，而是用于染料敏化太阳能电池这一能源领域。正因为如此，我工作初期的很大一部分工作内容就是能源材料的开发与应用，还为此专门与中国科学院物理研究所的陈立泉院士等 10 余人组队到欧洲参加中欧能源会议，并访问了染料敏化太阳能电池的开创人 Gratzel 教授的实验室（2004 年底）。

另一方面，作为一名年轻的新同事，我开始在工作中与崔老师有了较多的接触，这使我逐渐进入生物医用材料的领域。2004年工作伊始，崔老师就让我以孔祥东博士论文的工作为基础，申请了国家自然科学基金的青年基金项目——《丝素蛋白自组装调制生物矿化的研究》，这是我作为负责人申请到的第一个项目。在2004年第2届亚洲地区生物矿化研讨会前夕，崔老师积极推动我对博士工作做出总结，在会上做口头报告——*Formation of manganite fibers under the directing of cationic surfactant*，并因此认定我英语不错，于是相继让我担任了2004年10月在韩国首尔举办的中韩生物材料和纳米生物技术研讨会的中方秘书，以及2005年9月在青岛举办的第5届亚欧国际等离子体表面工程会议（简称为AEPSE2005）的大会秘书。2004年的中韩会议是我第一次出国，在此过程中我也结识了若干位时隔多年仍觉亲切的前辈同仁，包括延世大学的In-Seop Lee教授、华中科技大学的张胜民教授、北京大学口腔医院的冯海兰教授和中国医科大学附属口腔医院的赵宝红教授等。AEPSE2005国际会议也是我至今为止唯一一次担任大会秘书的会议，崔老师为此专门给我配备了我的第一台笔记本电脑。2005年8月，崔老师开始让我参与Myron Spector和他一起主持的哈佛-MIT-清华"组织工程学"网络课堂，由此结识了哈佛大学的Spector教授，这也成为我完全转入生物医用材料的一个契机（见后文）。

　　在2004—2006年这两年的工作中，我一直在能源材料与生物材料两个方向做工作，常感力不从心，想要确定一个方向深入下去。很长一段时间内，我的内心一直在纠结着自己的科研定向问题：两个都是热门的、有大发展前景的、对人类生活很有帮助的方向；太阳能电池材料是自己博士论文的延续，有背景，有基础；生物医用材料是自己在工作后才开始接触的，欠缺积累，但确是自己一直感兴趣的。最终，兴趣还是成为了我选择科研道路的主要因素。我决定出国深造，让自己学习更多生物医用材料相关的技术与知识。在与李先生和崔老师商谈后，他们都慷慨地答应帮我写推荐信。我于2006年8月作为国家留学基金管理委员会公派访问学者，到哈佛大学学习，在合作导师Myron Spector教授的研究组内开始了软骨组织工程工作的研究，从此完全进入了生物医用材料领域。访问学者的工作让我学习到了细胞培养、基因转染、组织切片等一些做生物医用材料所必需的知识，相应工作发表在*Biomaterials*上，还参加了材料研究协会年会、世界生物材料大会、国际组织工程与再生医学大会等一系列国际会议，可以说收获良多。

　　2007年8月回国后，我薄弱的生物医用材料基础让我只能想到延续软骨组织工程的研究工作。这时，崔老师同意我以他研制的矿化胶原仿生骨为基础，结合我在哈佛大学开展的软骨组织工程研究，制备骨软骨双相支架，其中，软骨区支架材料中所使用的水母来源胶原由东南大学钱卫平教授提供，这也是崔老师帮我介绍的功劳。通过与福建医科大学附属医院林建华院长的合作，与该双相支架相关的工作获得了福建省科技计划重点项目的支持，在 SCI 收录期刊发表文章，申请到一项专利。在这项研究工作的进展过程中，我又分别联系了中国人民解放军总医院的蔡胥主任和武警总医院的张仲文主任，学习了很多动物实验和临床病例的知识，为我深入生物医用材料的研究打下了一定的基础。但之后，由于确定品种的水母来源的缺失以及支架制备工艺时长的限制，学生们渐渐放下了这个方向的研究。

与此同时，由于我一直觉得人体里最奇妙的就是神经系统，所以一直希望自己能在神经领域做些事情。恰巧崔老师的博士生魏岳腾正在做透明质酸（hyaluronic acid，HA）用于脊髓损伤修复的工作，崔老师愿意魏岳腾多跟我交流，我便有机会接触到不少与神经支架材料相关的知识。在一次和魏岳腾交流的过程中，我了解到导电高分子材料用于神经组织工程的工作，这引起我很大的兴趣——与电相关的材料也许能利用到以前电池的相关工作吧？从 2007 年年底开始，我进行了大量有关聚吡咯（polypyrrole，PPy）及电信号对细胞作用的调研，并开始组织学生进行 PPy 的制备实验。2009 年，我有幸和崔老师一起（崔老师作为负责人，我作为主要执行人）与加拿大萨斯喀彻温大学的 Xiong-Biao Chen 申请到国家自然科学基金国际合作与交流项目——《用于脊髓损伤外科修复的生物工程支架研究》，这个项目里提出用 3D 打印方法制备 HA-PPy 框架材料。在完成这个项目的过程中，我接触并学习到很多 3D 打印技术及神经相关的知识，2011 年发表的综述文章 *Bioengineered scaffolds for spinal cord repair* 至今已被引用 21 次。另一方面，同样是通过崔老师的介绍，我结识了首都医科大学附属北京天坛医院的安沂华主任。出于对导电材料用于神经损伤修复的共同兴趣，安主任和我（我作为负责人）于 2010 年合作申请到北京市自然科学基金项目——《聚乳酸-纳米聚吡咯导电聚合物制备及培养间充质干细胞的研究》。在这个项目里，我们提出用溶剂挥发法制备聚乳酸（polylactic acid，PLA）/PPy 复合导电材料，用于骨髓间充质干细胞和脐带间充质干细胞的生长与分化研究。后来，我又进一步想知道支架的纤维微观形貌和电信号的共同作用会怎样影响干细胞的分化，于是开始以电纺方法制备 PLA/PPy 复合导电纤维膜。恰好本组的王秀梅教授也在用电纺方法制备水凝胶纤维材料用于神经损伤修复的研究，我们（我作为负责人）便于 2013 年合作申请到了两岸清华自主科研项目——《不同物化性能的定向电纺材料对干细胞的影响及机制研究》。最近，学生终于从聚合酯链式反应和蛋白荧光染色结果中证实了，我们的电纺 PLA/PPyPLA/PPy 复合导电纤维膜具有促进脐带间充质干细胞向神经细胞分化的作用。虽然现在相关文章还没能总结出来，但从研究 PPy 至今 8 年有余，经过几届学生的努力，终于克服了重重困难，让我看到了自己坚持一个研究方向后的曙光，这对我来讲不能不说是个极大的安慰。

2012 年，我在参加一次学校组织的教学研讨会时，无意中听工程物理系一位老师谈到他们在做核磁共振成像的工作中会用到纳米颗粒造影剂，我立刻想到，做纳米颗粒是我们的强项啊！于是，我先安排了一名做本科毕业设计的学生进行了最简单的制备氧化铁颗粒工作，并招收到颜昊这名成熟、有想法的研究生在这个领域上展开了一些比较深入的研究工作，同时把 PPy 拓展到光热治疗肿瘤的应用上。机缘巧合的是，在肿瘤诊疗方面有丰富经验的赵凌云老师于 2014 年底从工程物理系转到我们组，刚好把纳米颗粒材料应用于肿瘤诊疗的工作迅速推动起来。在 2015 年的生物材料研究组秋季学期第二次学术研讨会上，我的 3 位学生的工作汇报都展示出不错的结果，获得了本组老师们的一致好评。虽然我知道这距离我们获得国内外同仁的认可还有很大的距离，但是看到自己及学生们这几年下来的工作积累及进步时，我终于敢说：我是真的进入生物医用材料领域了。

对我来讲，转入生物医用材料的研究本就是个艰难而缓慢的过程，而我在回国后不久，就因各种原因，进入了一个工作发展缓慢期。等我再次回归到工作中时才发现，几年的蛰伏着实让我落下了不少工作，再加上我本就薄弱的科研基础，这两年的工作回归可以说是"拼得吃力"，尤其是拿项目和发文章的压力，让我中途几次升起"不干了，干不了"的念头。幸运的是，这期间很多人和事都在一直提醒我：做事情没有那么一帆风顺、轻轻松松的，一路的风风雨雨都能克服了、走下去，才会走出自己的一片天地。这些人和事中就包括崔老师从大学教授逐渐转到公司运营领域。我最近跟人谈起此事，最爱说的一句话就是：崔老师能这样跨界运作，能力是一方面，坚持与毅力真的是很重要的另一方面！

最近，崔老师又在尽力帮组内的年轻老师们寻找和提供一些加入"十三五"项目的机会，并总在国内同仁面前对我不吝称赞，这无疑也成为督促我坚持做下去，并努力做好的孜孜动力。

除了科研上的帮助，崔老师留给我印象最深的一件事就是，2011 年初，在我产假期间，他专门到我家里给我的宝宝送了一份红包和一件红色 T 恤，这让我感到充满惊喜的温暖——说话常常严厉不留情面的崔老师原来也有这么细腻温情的一面。

藉崔老师 70 岁生日之际，组内毕业的学生们再次欢聚一堂，并组织编写了这本书稿。熟人相见及阅读书稿之际，我深感自己获得了一次回顾清华大学材料科学与工程系生物材料研究组发展历程的机会，而我自己也在工作近 12 年之时，写下这篇文章，总结自己的工作发展历程，看到了知识积累、认真投入与同行合作的并重性，同时也再次理清了自己的科研道路选择：兴趣与坚持！

谨以此文表达我对崔老师提供各种机会与帮助的感谢之意！

# 2.9 您的指导和帮助如春雨
## ——献给崔福斋教授 70 岁生日

### 李晓明

北京航空航天大学，北京

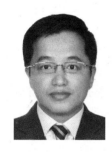

李晓明，北京航空航天大学教授、博士生导师。入选北京市科技新星计划、教育部新世纪优秀人才支持计划，获霍英东教育基金会高等院校青年教师基金。从事生物材料研究。

　　我于 2002 年 9 月进入崔老师负责的清华大学生物材料研究组攻读博士学位。尽管崔老师不是我的直接导师（冯庆玲教授），但是崔老师十几年来一直像导师一样指导、支持和帮助我。到目前为止，已共同在 SCI 收录期刊上发表文章 25 篇，SCI 引用 1 000 余次，其中 SCI 引用 55 次以上的有 7 篇。

　　众所周知，读博是宽进严出，尤其是清华大学材料科学与工程专业博士毕业要求相对较高，然而我是幸运的，除了获得导师冯老师的悉心指导之外，崔老师也给予了多方面的指导和帮助，使得我能够在读博期间研究出一种性能优良的新型三维多孔胶原基纤维增强骨组织工程支架材料——纳米晶羟基磷灰石/胶原/聚-L-乳酸/甲壳素纤维。该材料在结构和成分两方面均与天然骨相似；材料的多孔性与松质骨类似；甲壳素纤维的加入不但中和了聚-L-乳酸的酸性降解产物，而且还大大提高了材料的力学性能；并首次提出纤维增强三维多孔生物材料强度与纤维强度、长度、在材料中的体积含量的关系公式，为纤维增强材料的生物医用研究提供了一定的理论基础。该材料植入体内后，能与宿主骨胶原末端的氨基或羟基结合，形成具有生物活性的化学结合界面，使该材料本身就具备与骨键合的能力，不但能维持细胞正常表型表达，而且能激活细胞的特异基因表达。用该支架材料成功修复了长为 40 mm 的山羊腿节段性骨缺损。成果发表时，国内外尚未有用组织工程的方法成功修复长为 30 mm 以上的节段性骨缺损的报道。代表性文章 *Collagen-based implants reinforced by chitin fibres in a goat shank bone defect model* 发表于期刊 *Biomaterials* 上，列该期刊 "Top 50 Highly Cited Articles By Chinese Mainland Authors 2006—2010"，SCI 引用不少于 100 次。基于在胶原基骨修复材料方面的研究成果，我和崔老师被邀请为著作 *Biomaterials and Regenerative Medicine*（主编为密歇根大学的 Peter X. Ma 教授）撰写题为 *Collagen based tissue repair composite* 的一章，该著作已由剑桥大学出版社出版。

在二位导师的悉心指导下，我攻读博士学位比较顺利，以第一作者发表 6 篇 SCI 文章，于 2005 年 11 月完成学位论文答辩。但是，毕业后又面临一个新的难题——就业或者去向问题。非常感谢崔老师推荐我去了荷兰特文特大学做博士后，之后又推荐我申获了日本学术振兴会（Japan Society for the Promotion of Science，JSPS）研究员的工作，到日本北海道大学工作。在国外学习和工作的 3 年中，崔老师不断通过电子邮件给予指导。当时，荷兰研究组的一项主要工作是磷酸钙陶瓷用做骨修复材料的研究。通过动物实验，他们发现某些磷酸钙陶瓷能够在软组织中诱导成骨。但是，为什么这些材料具有这种骨诱导性一直未得到合理解释。为了揭示该骨诱导机制，我们制备了多种微结构相同、成分不同以及成分相同、微结构不同的磷酸钙陶瓷，并通过多种骨关联细胞与其共培养以及后续的大量生化实验发现，由于具有骨诱导性的磷酸钙陶瓷具有独特的微结构，因此有能力吸附大量的特定成骨关联蛋白，这些被吸附的成骨关联蛋白最终在软组织中诱导成骨，并通过结构分析与计算，提出了具有骨诱导性的磷酸钙陶瓷材料微结构与某些特定成骨关联蛋白分子结构之间的相关性模型。该机制的提出对成骨活性优良的磷酸钙陶瓷乃至其他骨修复材料的设计和研发具有重要的指导意义。代表性文章 *The effect of calcium phosphate micro-structure on bone-related cells in vitro* 发表于期刊 *Biomaterials* 上，SCI 引用不少于 141 次。期刊 *Biomaterials* 对该文初稿的评审意见为 "the referees advise that it should be accepted without scientific revision"。

日本学术振兴会研究员的工作结束后，我又是在崔老师的支持和帮助下进入北京航空航天大学工作，到目前为止，已在本单位工作满 6 年。回国后，崔老师反复对我强调，要结合国外的基础和本单位的条件做有特色的工作。目前，越来越多的纳米材料用于生物医用。具有代表性之一的碳纳米管（carbon nanotube，CNT）由于其独特的性能，正受到越来越多的关注。我通过先后主持国家自然科学基金项目（31000431）、北京市科技新星计划（2010B011）、教育部新世纪优秀人才支持计划（NCET-11-0769）等在国内较早地开展了 CNT 用做骨修复材料的系统研究。通过对 CNT 在体外和体内的系统研究发现：纯 CNT 经过一定改性后能够促进多种细胞（包括脂肪干细胞）向成骨质方向分化；改性后的 CNT 能够在骨缺损部位和某些软组织内直接或间接促进骨组织生成，在一定条件下还能够促进脊髓组织再生。这些研究为 CNT 能够用做生物活性骨修复材料提供了重要依据。此外，还研发出一类性能优良的含有 CNT 的三维多孔骨修复材料。代表性文章 *The use of carbon nanotubes to induce osteogenic differentiation of human adipose-derived MSCs in vitro and ectopic bone formation in vivo* 发表于本研究领域顶尖期刊 *Biomaterials* 上，发表后 3 年内，SCI 引用不少于 107 次，列 ESI 近 10 年高被引用文章。并且在期刊 *Journal of Biomedical Materials Research Part A* 上发表一篇相关综述文章 *Nanostructured scaffolds for bone tissue engineering*，发表后两年内，SCI 引用不少于 83 次，列 ESI 近 10 年高被引用文章。

总之，我成长的每一步都离不开崔老师的教诲、指导和大力支持。恭祝崔老师 70 岁生日快乐、身体健康、福如东海、寿比南山！

# 共同发表的代表性文章

1. Li X M, Feng Q L, Liu X H, Dong W, Cui F Z. Collagen-based implants reinforced by chitin fibres in a goat shank bone defect model. *Biomaterials*, 2006, 27 (9)：1917-1923.

**Abstract**　Tissue engineering is an increasingly popular method for repairing bone defects. However, repair of bone defects over 30 mm using tissue-engineering methods is a difficult clinical problem. In this study, we used a goat shank model to evaluate the bone-regenerating efficacy of a novel nano-hydroxyapatite/collagen/PLLA (nHACP) composite reinforced by chitin fibres. Forty adult male goats with 40 mm defects in shank at the same anatomic site were divided into four groups. The first group was the control, where nothing was implanted in the defect (defect group). The other three groups were implanted with porous pure PLLA, nHACP and nHACP reinforced by chitin fibres, respectively. Bone growth in each group was evaluated by radiography, histology, bone mineral density and mechanical strength, once every 5 weeks for 15 weeks. The results indicated that nHACP implants, both with and without chitin fibres, are better for repairing the defects than pure PLLA. However, only the reinforced implants showed nearly perfect recovery in 15 weeks after operation. So, the reinforced scaffold might be a candidate for bone tissue repair.

引用次数：**100**

2. Li X M, van Blitterswijk C A, Feng Q L, Cui F Z, Watari F. The effect of calcium phosphate microstructure on bone-related cells in vitro. *Biomaterials*, 2008, 29 (23)：3306-3316.

**Abstract**　Microstructure is essential for inductive bone formation in calcium phosphate materials after soft tissue implantation. We hereby evaluated activities (cell attachment, proliferation, ALP/DNA and protein/DNA) of three types of cells cultured on three kinds of calcium phosphate ceramic discs to study how microstructure takes its role in inductive bone formation. Three kinds of biphasic calcium phosphate (BCP) ceramic discs with the same chemistry and the same dimension of circle divide $\phi10.0\times1.0$ mm$^3$ (BCP1150-P, BCP1150-D and BCP1300), either having similar micropore sizes and surface roughness but different surface area (BCP1150-P vs BCP1150-D) or having similar surface area but different micropore sizes and different roughness (BCP1150-D vs BCP1300), were prepared. Conventionally Culturing C2C12, human bone marrow stromal cells (HBMSC) and MC3T3-E1 cells on BCP discs showed that, surface roughness did not affect cell attachment, cell proliferation and ALP expression of all cell types evaluated, while surface area did affect cell functions. ALP/DNA of C2C12 on BCP1150-P, having larger surface area, was significantly higher than on BCP1300 and BCP1150-D. Furthermore, all cells cultured on all of the three kinds of BCPs pre-soaked in culture medium having additional rhBMP-2 had a higher ALP expression than the conventional cell culture. Comparing with on BCP1300 and BCP1150-D, ALP/DNA of all cells tested increased more on BCP1150-P after the discs were pre-soaked in culture medium with rhBMP-2. The results indicated that increasing surface areas, microstructured calcium phosphate materials might concentrate more proteins (including bone-inducing proteins) that differentiate inducible cells to osteogenic cells that form inductive bone.

引用次数: **141**

3. Li X M, Liu H F, Niu X F, Yu B, Fan Y B, Feng Q L, Cui F Z, Watari F. The use of carbon nanotubes to induce osteogenic differentiation of human adipose-derived MSCs in vitro and ectopic bone formation in vivo. *Biomaterials*, 2012, 33 (19): 4818-4827.

**Abstract** Carbon nanotubes (CNTs), one of the most concerned nanomaterials, with unique electrical, mechanical and surface properties, have been shown suitable for biomedical application. In this study, we evaluated attachment, proliferation, osteogenic gene expression, ALP/DNA, protein/DNA and mineralization of human adipose-derived stem cells cultured in vitro on multi-walled carbon nanotubes (MWNTs) and graphite (GP) compacts with the same dimension. Moreover, we assessed the effect of these two kinds of compacts on ectopic bone formation in vivo. First of all, higher ability of the MWNTs compacts to adsorb proteins, comparing with the GP compacts, was shown. During the conventional culture, it was shown that

MWNTs could induce the expression of ALP, cbfa1 and COLIA1 genes while GP could not. Furthermore, alkaline phosphatase (ALP)/DNA and protein/DNA of the cell on the MWNTs compacts, was significantly higher than those of the cells on the GP compacts. With the adsorption of the proteins in culture medium with 50% fetal bovine serum (FBS) in advance, the increments of the ALP/DNA and protein/DNA for the MWNTs compacts were found respectively significantly more than the increments of those for the GP compacts, suggesting that the larger amount of protein adsorbed on the MWNTs was crucial. More results showed that ALP/DNA and protein/DNA of the cells on the two kinds of compacts pre-soaked in culture medium having additional rhBMP-2 were both higher than those of the cells on the samples re-soaked in culture medium with 50% FBS, and that those values for the MWNTs compacts increased much more. Larger mineral content was found on the MWNTs compacts than on the GP compacts at day 7. In vivo experiment showed that the MWNTs could induce ectopic bone formation in the dorsal musculature of ddy mice while GP could not. The results indicated that MWNTs might stimulate inducible cells in soft tissues to form inductive bone by concentrating more proteins, including bone-inducing proteins.

引用次数: **107**

4. Li X M, Wang L, Fan Y B, Feng Q L, Cui F Z, Watari F. Nanostructured scaffolds for bone tissue engineering. *Journal of Biomedical Materials Research Part A*, 2013, 101A (8): 2424-2435.

**Abstract**　It has been demonstrated that nanostructured materials, compared with conventional materials, may promote greater amounts of specific protein interactions, thereby more efficiently stimulating new bone formation. It has also been indicated that, when features or ingredients of scaffolds are nanoscaled, a variety of interactions can be stimulated at the cellular level. Some of those interactions induce favorable cellular functions while others may leads to toxicity. This review presents the mechanism of interactions between nanoscaled materials and cells and focuses on the current research status of nanostructured scaffolds for bone tissue engineering. Firstly, the main requirements for bone tissue engineering scaffolds were discussed. Then, the mechanism by which nanoscaled materials promote new bone formation was explained, following which the current research status of main types of nanostructured scaffolds for bone tissue engineering was reviewed and discussed.

引用次数: **83**

# 第三部分

## 曾经的学生畅谈科研创新

# 3.1 仿生合成骨缺损修复材料研究的回顾和一点体会

杜　昶

华南理工大学材料科学与工程学院，广州

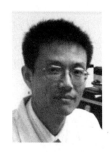

杜昶，华南理工大学材料科学与工程学院教授，教育部创新团队负责人。1994 年，于清华大学材料科学与工程系获学士学位；1999 年，于清华大学材料科学与工程系获材料物理与化学专业博士学位，师从崔福斋教授，研究天然骨微结构及仿生复合骨替代材料；2002 年，于荷兰莱顿大学医学院获得博士学位，师从 Klaas de Groot 教授，研究利用仿生技术对可降解生物高分子材料进行表面改性并应用于骨组织工程；2003—2008 年，在美国南加利福尼亚大学颅面分子生物学中心先后从事博士后研究及担任研究助理，在 Janet Moradian-Oldak 教授的研究组从事牙釉质生物矿化研究，首次建立釉原蛋白分级自组装过程模型，揭示牙釉质生物矿化机理，作为第一作者的文章发表在 Science 上，获得国际学术界广泛关注。研究领域包括生物矿化与仿生、生物医用材料和组织工程。

　　1994 年，我幸运地获得直博资格并成为崔福斋教授的第一届博士研究生，从此步入生物材料领域的科学殿堂，主要研究骨、牙齿等天然硬组织的生物矿化特性及用于修复缺损组织的仿生型材料。5 年博士研究生的历练，为我日后的科研工作打下了坚实的基础。当年实验室里的点点滴滴仍历历在目，从选题到具体的科研实践，从对研究结果的分析整理到文章的撰写，崔老师对国际研究前沿的敏锐把握及其广泛而活跃的创新思维，对我的科研启蒙乃至今后的职业发展都产生了不可磨灭的深远影响。如今，我自己也已成为一名教师和研究生导师，不仅为研究生开设生物矿化方面的专业课程，也在指导 10 余名研究生开展科研。崔老师的教导仍然在不经意间贯穿于我和学生的互动之中，而博士期间形成的学术思想更是在我的科研实践中发挥着重要作用。

　　应用于骨和牙齿等硬组织缺损修复和替代的材料是生物医学材料中的一大

类，临床需求量大，涉及面广。然而，相比作为骨修复"金标准"的自体骨移植，各种人工材料仍然存在很多局限。我一进入实验室，崔老师便指导我在磷酸钙–胶原仿生自体骨的骨修复材料研究方向上深入探索，并要求我详细掌握国内外的研究动态，特别是最近10年内的相关进展，这样才能发现当前尚未解决的关键问题。这也是他从其导师李恒德先生处得到的治学经验。经过充分调研，我发现当时磷酸钙–胶原复合材料的研究总体上还比较初步，材料的复合大多是采用传统磷酸钙生物陶瓷和胶原的机械混合方法，利用了磷酸钙陶瓷良好的生物活性和骨传导性，而胶原提供了使陶瓷颗粒分散分布的框架，并将这些颗粒粘接在一起。这类混合物在成分上与骨组织相似，但其组织反应和传统的磷酸钙类生物陶瓷没有本质上的差别，例如，高温烧结的羟基磷灰石陶瓷颗粒在胶原降解后仍能长期存在，陶瓷与胶原基体之间无法形成紧密的键合，陶瓷颗粒只能松散的分布于胶原框架内，并未真正解决使用传统生物陶瓷所碰到的问题。事实上，骨作为一种天然生物复合材料，在成分及结构上均具有一些独特的特征，发展成分和结构均高度仿生自体骨的骨修复材料还面临很大的挑战。幸运的是，崔老师的研究组已经开始从仿生矿化的角度，通过体外模拟骨组织在体内的矿化过程发展新型材料，并已有初步成果，但关于这类新型仿生材料与细胞和组织的相互作用还不清楚。这方面的深入研究无疑将为更好地设计、制造与应用该类材料打下基础。我的博士课题因此确定下来，一方面进一步探索磷酸钙–胶原复合材料的仿生制备方法，另一方面深入研究这些材料与细胞和生物组织的相互作用，并与骨组织工程学结合开展基础研究，具体包括利用大鼠肌袋模型和小鼠腹腔巨噬细胞体外培养模型研究材料的生物降解性能；利用兔股骨骨髓腔内植入模型研究复合材料的成骨性能和体内的降解行为；以及根据组织工程学原理构建成骨性细胞与复合材料支架的三维复合体的研究等。这些研究取得了很好的成果，3篇代表性文章都发表在当时生物材料领域的重要期刊 *Journal of Biomedical Materials Research* 上，得到了同行的广泛关注。目前，单篇引用次数分别为194次、210次和276次。这些文章的摘要见文后。

基于有机基质调制仿生矿化的思想，我们将胶原片在高 pH 值和高 $PO_4^{3-}$ 离子浓度的溶液中处理，使其成为高度负电性的基质，随后在含 $Ca^{2+}$ 离子溶液中反应，$Ca^{2+}$ 离子向基质内的快速扩散导致了矿物的迅速沉积。胶原的负电性基团与 $Ca^{2+}$ 离子之间存在较强的静电相互作用，因此，经去离子水反复冲洗后，钙化胶原片仍保持了较高的矿物含量，可占总质量的 60%～70%。复合材料的力学性能指标达到了骨的力学性能数据的下限，抗拉强度为 6.08～11 MPa，杨氏模量为 0.66～2.24 GPa。

当将仿生制备的具有纳米晶特征的磷酸钙–胶原复合材料用于修复兔股骨缺损，结果显示这种模仿了骨的成分与微结构特征的复合材料具有优异的生物活性，同时具有良好的生物可降解性能。一方面材料支持新生骨组织在其表面上生长，另一方面材料通过溶液或细胞介导的过程被机体降解，组织学形态的表现非常类似骨组织本身的生理性重构过程。这些发现预示了这种仿生材料有可能通过机体自身的新陈代谢而被整合进入组织的再生修复过程中。

利用所制备的片状复合材料具有较好的柔韧性的特点，我们结合组织细胞培养技术并将片状材料卷成具有适宜尺寸的三维多孔支架，从而使细胞在三维支架中均匀分布。支架的多孔结构具有几十至几百微米大小的孔隙，有利于细胞的贴附和生长，并可以提供充足的空间促进营养的输送、血管和骨组织等的长入。这种由仿生骨支架装载具成骨能力的细胞构成的三维复合体有望在骨缺损的修复中发挥作用。

Wojciech L. Suchanek 等在其文章（*Biomaterials*，2002，23：699-710）中引用上述工作并进行了积极评价，肯定了仿生合成的低结晶度和纳米尺度的磷灰石在制备类骨材料方面的重要性：

"Nanosized $CO_3HAp$ crystals were successfully applied to fabricate $CO_3HAp$/collagen biodegradable composites. When implanted in rabbits, these materials underwent resorption and promoted new bone formation." "$CO_3HAp$ powders with low crystallinity and nanometer particle size are suitable for the processing of bone-resembling materials."

Guo-Bao Wei 和 Peter X. Ma 在综述性文章（*Adv. Funct. Mater.*，2008，18：3568-3582）中也引用了上述工作：

"To mimic the nanofeatures of natural bone, collagen/nano-HAp（nHAp）composite or porous composite matrices were fabricated by precipitation of HAp nanoparticles from an aqueous solution onto collagen. Interfacial new bone formation by osteoblasts was observed after implantation in a rabbit marrow cavity. Biodegradation of the composite was achieved by solution-mediated dissolution and possibly cell mediated resorption in which the nanometer size of HAp particles was important"

并且，他们认为这类材料提供了与体内环境相类似的微环境，从而有助于骨组织的再生：

"The results suggest that the porous collagen/nHAp scaffold may provide a microenvironment similar to in vivo environment favorable for bone regeneration."

Karen J. L. Burg 等学者在关于骨组织工程支架材料的综述性文章中（*Biomaterials*，2000，21：2347-2359）详细介绍了我们利用卷绕的方法构建细胞与多孔支架三维复合体的工作：

"Du and coworkers have demonstrated that collagen sheets can be used as the basis for composite bone tissue-engineering scaffolds. Du obtained commercially available collagen sheets, precipitated HA onto the surface, then placed bone fragments along the surface, rolling the composite into a tube. The pore sizes in this material range from tens to hundreds of microns; the material is absorbable and flexible. Cells migrated from the bone fragments into the matrix, suggesting that the material is bioactive. "

上述工作多年来受到持续关注，如 Zeng-Ming Xia 等在近期的文章（*Acta Biomaterialia*，2013，9：7308-7319）中引用了上述文章。又如 A. Ronca 等发表的文章（*Acta Biomaterialia*，2013，9：5989-5996）所进行的引用和评述，肯定了模仿天然骨的成分和微结构所构建的仿生材料对提高缺损组织的修复效果具有重要的积极作用。

"Orthopaedic research suggests that osteoconductivity would be optimal when synthetic HAp resembles the bone mineral with regard to composition, size and morphology. " "Well-dispersed nanosized hydroxyapatite (nano-HAp) with an ultrafine structure has the potential to improve the performance of composites, because these particles have a high surface area to volume ratio and their surfaces have minimal defects. "

这些早期的创新性工作也为我之后的科研打下了很好的基础。例如，在人工合成高聚物聚乙二醇（polyethylene glycol，PEG）/聚对苯二甲酸丁二醇酯（polybutylene terephthalate，PBT）表面仿生沉积类骨羟基磷灰石涂层，动物实验表明，仿生涂层可提高 PEG/PBT 材料的生物活性，促进植入物与骨组织的整合；应用仿生合成技术在钛金属表面制备牙釉质蛋白与磷灰石的复合材料涂层，利用体外细胞培养技术研究材料与间充质成骨细胞前体的相互作用，发现新型涂层对细胞在骨特异性基因的表达中具有显著的增强作用。

目前，仿生合成骨缺损修复材料的研究已成为重要的国际研究前沿。当然，相关的研究已经不仅限于利用仿生合成技术制备出与天然骨相类似的成分和纳米晶体结构。根据本人的了解和近几年的实践，将仿生技术与其他制造技术结合获得可调控多级孔结构或多级结构的复合支架材料，是当前和未来研究的一个重要内容。

天然骨组织具有从纳米到厘米的分级结构，其增强和增韧机制不仅由于有机和无机组分的存在，而且很大程度上得益于多尺度的分级结构；此外，骨中矿物相不是离散的磷酸钙晶体的聚集，而是以连续相形式存在，这对骨的力学性能也是很重要的。对天然骨及其他生物矿化材料的多级结构和性能的深入认识仍旧是富有挑战的研究方向。

此外，利用仿生合成技术有可能获得具有独特特征和性能的材料，例如，具有较高比表面积的微纳米颗粒，将这些材料作为载体负载细胞、药物、基因、微 RNA 等，并研究其效果和所出现的新规律都是近几年的热点方向。

# 培养期间代表性文章

1. Du C, Cui F Z, Zhu X D, de Groot K. Three-dimensional nano-HAp/collagen matrix loading with osteogenic cells in organ culture. *Journal of Biomedical Materials Research*, 1999, 44 (4): 407-415.

**Abstract**    Transplantation of osteogenic cells with a suitable matrix is one strategy for engineering bone tissue. Three-dimensional distribution and growth of cells within the porous scaffold are of clinical significance for the repair of large bony defects. A nano-HAp/collagen (nHAC) composite that mimics the natural bone both in composition and microstructure to some extent was employed as a matrix for the tissue engineering of bone. A porous nHAC composite was produced in sheet form and convolved to be a three-dimensional scaffold. Using organ culture techniques and the convolving method, we have developed three-dimensional osteogenic cells/nHAC constructs in vitro. Scanning electron microscopic and histological examination has demonstrated the development of the cells/material complex. Spindle-shaped cells migrating out of bone fragments continuously proliferated and migrated throughout the network of the coil. The porous nHAC scaffold provided a microenvironment resembling that seen in vivo, and cells within the composite eventually acquired a tridimensional polygonal shape. In addition, new bone matrix was synthesized at the interface of bone fragments and the composite.

引用次数: **282**

2. Du C, Cui F Z, Zhang W, Feng Q L, Zhu X D, de Groot K. Formation of calcium phosphate/collagen composites through mineralization of collagen matrix. *Journal of Biomedical Materials Research*, 2000, 50 (4): 518-527.

**Abstract**    Several types of calcium phosphate/collagen composites, including noncrystalline calcium phosphate/collagen, poorly crystalline carbonate-apatite (PCCA)/collagen, and PCCA + tetracalcium phosphate/collagen composites, were prepared through the mineralization of collagen matrix. The type I collagen was presoaked with a $PO_4^{3-}$ containing solution and then immersed in a $Ca^{2+}$ containing solution to allow mineral deposition. The solution of 0.56M sodium dibasic phosphate ($Na_2HPO_4$) with a pH of nearly 14 was metastable and its crystallization produced $Na_2HPO_4$ and sodium tripolyphosphate hexahydrate ($Na_5P_3O_{10} \cdot 6H_2O$), leading to a controlled release of orthophosphate ions during the subsequent mineral precipitation. The development of the composites was investigated in detail. The mineral contributed up to 60 - 70% of the weight of the final composites. The strength and

Young's modulus of the composites in tensile tests overlapped the lower range of values reported for bone. When implanted in muscle tissue, the composite showed biodegradability that was partly through a multinucleated giant cell mediated process. In a bone explant culture model it was observed that bone-derived cells deposited mineralizing collagenous matrix on the composite.

引用次数: **188**

3. Du C, Cui F Z, Feng Q L, Zhu X D, de Groot K. Tissue response to nano-hydroxyapatite/collagen composite implants in marrow cavity. *Journal of Biomedical Materials Research*, 1998, 42 (4): 540-548.

**Abstract**  The tissue response to a nano-hydroxyapatite/collagen composite implanted in a marrow cavity was investigated by histology and scanning electron microscopy. A Knoop microhardness test was performed to compare the mechanical behavior of the composite and bone. The ultrastructural features of the composite, especially the carbonate-substituted hydroxyapatite with low crystallinity and nanometer size, made it a bone-resembling material. It was bioactive, as well as biodegradable. At the interface of the implant and marrow tissue, solution-mediated dissolution and giant cell mediated resorption led to the degradation of the composite. Interfacial bone formation by osteoblasts was also evident. The process of implant degradation and bone substitution was reminiscent of bone remodeling. The composite can be incorporated into bone metabolism instead of being a permanent implant. For lack of the hierarchical organization similar to that of bone, the composite exhibited an isotropic mechanical behavior. However, the resistance of the composite to localized pressure could reach the lower limit of that of the femur compacta.

引用次数: **166**

4. Du C, Su X W, Cui F Z, Zhu X D. Morphological behaviour of osteoblasts on diamond-like carbon coating and amorphous C−N film in organ culture. *Biomaterials*, 1998, 19 (7-9): 651-658.

**Abstract**  Similar to diamond-like carbon (DLC) coating, amorphous carbon nitride (C−N) films can be extremely hard and wear-resistant. They may serve as candidates for the solution to the problem of aseptic loosening of total hip replacements. Morphological behaviour of osteoblasts on silicon, DLC-coated silicon and amorphous C−N film-deposited silicon in organ culture was investigated by scanning electron microscopy. Cells on the silicon wafers were able to attach, but were unable to follow this attachment with spreading. In contrast, the cells attached, spread and proliferated on the DLC coatings and amorphous C−N films without apparent impairment of cell physiology. The morphological development of cells on the coatings and films was similar to that of cells in the control. The preliminary results support the biocompatibility of DLC coating and are encouraging for the potential biomedical applications of amorphous C−N film.

引用次数: 97

# 3.2　Letter from Hai-Bo Wen

Hai-Bo Wen

Director of Research, Dental, Zimmer Biomet

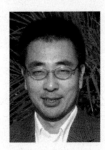

Hai Bo Wen, Zimmer Biomet Dental 科研主管，负责领导全球科研和临床事务部门。分别于 1992 年和 1995 年在清华大学材料科学与工程系获材料科学学士学位和材料物理学硕士学位；1998 年，在荷兰莱顿大学获生物材料学博士学位。在生物矿化、生物材料、表面改性以及组织再生在骨科、脊柱和牙科中的应用领域有着 20 年的研发经验。

In early 1990s, scientists in the materials science and engineering field realized that mother of nature has taught us a lot of lessons in synthesizing strong and tough mineralized tissues, such as bone, dentin, tooth enamel, nacre, and ivory tusk etc. Prof. Heng-De Li and Prof. Cui were among the pioneers who started researching the ultra-structure of natural hard tissues and using the underlying principles to design novel composite materials for clinical and various industrial applications. I was recruited as one of their first graduate students to conduct additional research in these areas.

I was greatly indebted to Prof. Cui for his fine teaching during my college years and gracious support to my joint Ph. D. program between Tsinghua University and Leiden University. During the graduate school years (1992—1998), he provided me critical guidance on how to conduct and publish scientific research and led me into the wonderland of biological materials. We realized how much a material scientist can learn from the mother of nature.

The first part of my Ph. D. program was focusing on the characterizations of ivory tusk, dental enamel and fracture healing callus. Prof. Cui guided me through the basic steps of doing research and writing English manuscripts for publications in peer-reviewed scientific journals. In order to familiarize myself with relevant medical literature, I made numerous trips to the central library of Beijing city and the libraries of surrounding dental and medical schools. The early collaborations with dental and orthopedic clinicians, such as Dr. Xiang-Qun Chen and Dr. Qing Wang and Dr. Xiao-Dong Zhu, had also helped to improve our understandings of medical procedures and patient needs.

This early phase of scientific research and exposure to biology and medicine prepared me well for the continuation of Ph. D. program in Leiden University, The Netherlands. My Ph. D. advisor there, Prof. Klaas de Groot was one of the pioneers in applying plasma sprayed hydroxyapatite coating on orthopedic and dental implants. He had the vision of developing a calcium phosphate coating for metallic implant with a biomimetic approach. Inspired by the biomineralization process of natural hard tissues, I was able to find ways to grow calcium phosphate crystals on titanium substrates. Some of the results were published in *Journal of Crystal Growth* (Vol. 186, pages 616-623, 1998). This so called biomimetic calcium phosphate coating can also be used as vehicle for incorporating and/or delivering therapeutic agents.

Various forms of calcium phosphate coatings have been commercialized for dental and orthopedic applications due to their superior biocompatibility and bone integration capability. Nowadays, a hydroxyapatite coating is still being considered as a gold standard for evaluating new surface modification techniques for improving bone integration.

The strong influences from Prof. Cui and later Prof. Klaas de Groot have set my research and professional life on a path in the medical device industry and that has not changed over the past 15 years: 5 years with DePuy, a Johnson and Johnson Company, 2 years with Calcitec, Inc. (a startup company developing spine fusion products) and 8 years with Zimmer's biology and dental divisions.

It was a pity to miss Prof. Cui's 70th birthday celebration. I was caught up in recent months by the post-merger integration of Zimmer Biomet and my family's move from Carlsbad, California to West Palm Beach, Florida. Turning into middle age myself now, I realized that Prof. Cui is one of very few individuals who have made significant impact to my life.

Congratulations to Prof. Cui for his professional accomplishments and remarkable contributions to many scientific research areas, such as materials physics, biomineralization, biomimetics, biomaterials and tissue engineering, etc. At his 70th birthday, I sincerely wish him and his family well and believe that his marvelous accomplishments will surely be followed by many successes in the coming decades.

## 培养期间代表性文章

1. Wen H B, Wolke J G C, de Wijn J R, Liu Q, Cui F Z, de Groot K. Fast

precipitation of calcium phosphate layers on titanium induced by simple chemical treatments. *Biomaterials*, 1997, 18 (22): 1471-1478.

**Abstract** A simple two-step chemical treatment, i. e. etching with HCl and $H_2SO_4$ followed by immersion in boiling dilute NaOH solution, has been developed by our group to prepare bioactive microporous titanium surfaces allowing fast deposition of a calcium phosphate layer (CPL) from an in vitro supersaturated calcification solution (SCS). In this work, a precalcification (Pre-Ca) procedure was applied by soaking the two-step treated titanium in $Na_2HPO_4$ and then saturated $Ca(OH)_2$ solution before immersion in SCS to accelerate further the CPL precipitation. The treated titanium surfaces with Pre-Ca were characterized after 1, 2, 4, 8 and 16 h of immersion in SCS by means of scanning electron microscopy together with energy dispersive X-ray analysis, X-ray diffraction and infrared absorption analysis. It was observed that the CPL precipitation rate with Pre-Ca averaged 1 $\mu$m h$^{-1}$ twice as fast as without Pre-Ca. No precipitation was observed on untreated titanium with Pre-Ca up to day 14 of immersion in the SCS.

引用次数: **132**

2. Wen H B, Liu Q, de Wijn J R, de Groot K, Cui F Z. Preparation of bioactive microporous titanium surface by a new two-step chemical treatment. *Journal of Materials Science: Materials in Medicine*, 1998, 9 (3): 121-128.

**Abstract** Microporous oxide layers allowing fast deposition of calcium phosphate layers (CPLs) were formed on commercially pure titanium (c. p. Ti) after the application of a newly developed two-step chemical treatment. The micropores were of submicrometre size. The two-step treatment was carried out by etching c. p. Ti samples with HCl and $H_2SO_4$ first and then treating them in boiling 0. 2 N NaOH solution at 140 ℃ for 5 h. Conformal CPLs, about 20 $\mu$m thick, were deposited on the two-step treated c. p. Ti surface by means of a two-day immersion in an in vitro supersaturated calcification solution. The CPL was characterized to be mainly composed of two sublayers, i. e. an outside loose octacalcium phosphate crystal sublayer and an inside dense carbonated apatite sublayer. A scratching test indicated that the apatite sublayer was strongly bonded to the c. p. Ti substrate. Moreover, it was observed that the untreated or single-step treated c. p. Ti surfaces are not only morphologically different from one another but significantly different from the two-step treated one, in that no precipitation was observed on them up to 14 d immersion in the same calcification solution. It is indicated that the two-step chemical treatment is a simple and easily controllable method to prepare bioactive titanium surfaces and subsequently to induce the rapid precipitation of conformal and adherent CPL from in vitro supersaturated calcification solutions.

3. Wen H B, de Wijn J R, Cui F Z, de Groot K. Preparation of calcium phosphate coatings on titanium implant materials by simple chemistry. *Journal of Biomedical Materials Research*, 1998, 41（2）: 227-236.

**Abstract**    A two-step chemical treatment has been developed in our group to prepare commercially pure titanium（cpTi）surfaces that will allow calcium phosphate（Ca-P）precipitation during immersion in a supersaturated calcification solution（SCS）with ion concentrations of $[Ca^{2+}] = 3.10$ mM and $[HPO_4^{2-}] = 1.86$ mM. It was observed that a precalcification（Pre-Ca）procedure prior to immersion could significantly accelerate the Ca-P deposition process. In this work, the bioactivity of chemically treated cpTi and Ti6Al4V was further verified by applying commercially available Hanks' balanced salt solution（HBSS）, an SCS with very low ion concentrations of $[Ca^{2+}] = 1.26$ mM and $[HPO_4^{2-}] = 0.779$ mM, as the immersion solution. It was found that a uniform and very dense apatite coating containing magnesium impurities was formed if the Pre-Ca procedure was performed before immersion, as compared with the loose Ca-P layer obtained from the abovementioned high concentration of SCS. The formation of a microporous titanium dioxide thin surface layer on cpTi or Ti6Al4V by the two-step chemical treatment could be the main reason for the induction of apatite nucleation and growth from HBSS. Variations of pH values, Ca and P concentrations, and immersion time in HBSS were investigated to reveal the detailed process of Ca-P deposition. The described treatments provide a simple chemical method to prepare Ca-P coatings on both cpTi and $Ti_6Al_4V$.

4. Wen H B, de Wijn J R, Cui F Z, de Groot K. Preparation of bioactive Ti6Al4V surfaces by a simple method. *Biomaterials*, 1998, 19（1-3）: 215-221.

**Abstract**    Boiling diluted alkali incubation was found to be an effective way to prepare bioactive Ti6Al4V surfaces, whether polished or not, as indicated in vitro after immersion in two different supersaturated calcification solutions（SCSs）. The induction of calcium phosphate（Ca-P）precipitation from the SCSs is most probably made possible by the formation of a new $TiO_2$ surface layer and a large number of submicron-scaled etched pits therein. The morphologies and composition of the Ca-P deposited from different SCSs are entirely different from each other. The processes on Ti6Al4V surfaces during treatment and immersion were investigated in detail by means of scanning electron microscopy combined with energy dispersive X-ray analysis, X-ray photoelectron spectroscopy and X-ray diffraction.

# 3.3　碳纳米材料的表面修饰及生物应用

李德军

天津师范大学物理与材料科学学院，天津

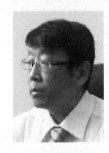

李德军，于清华大学获博士学位。现任天津师范大学物理所所长，物理系主任。从事材料-生物材料表面改性研究。

　　碳元素作为构成自然界物质基础的关键元素之一，作为人类认识最早的化学元素之一，在人类文明发展史中扮演着至关重要的角色，其独特的物理和化学性质与多样的形态总是随着人类科学文明的发展与进步而被逐渐认知。近20年来，碳纳米材料一直是纳米科技领域中的重要研究课题。1985年发现的富勒烯[1]（1996年被授予诺贝尔奖）、1991年发现的碳纳米管[2]和2004年首次制备出的石墨烯[3]（2010年被授予诺贝尔奖），已成为零维、一维和二维碳纳米材料的经典代表，均引发了世界范围的研究热潮。与其他的常规材料相比，碳纳米材料具有许多独特的效应：量子尺寸效应、微小尺寸效应、表面效应、量子隧道效应等。因此，碳纳米材料已经被广泛地应用到电化学、电催化、光学、生物材料、电子、分析器件以及储能器件等领域[4-6]。自1963年Gott在研究人工血管过程中发现碳具有较好的抗血栓性以来，碳材料已在人工心脏瓣膜、人工牙根、人工血管、人工骨与人工关节、人工韧带和肌腱等诸多方面获得临床应用。碳纳米材料除具有微米级碳纤维的低密度、高比强度、高比模量、高导电性之外，还具有缺陷数量极少、比表面积较大、结构致密等特点。由于碳纳米材料的这些超特性和它的良好生物相容性，使其在生物医学材料领域得到了广泛的关注和运用。

　　但是，随着对碳纳米材料生物医学应用研究的不断深入，碳纳米材料本身也暴露出一定的缺陷和问题。几乎所有的碳纳米材料都传承了天然石墨既不亲水也不亲油的性能，例如，原始状态下的碳纳米管是成千上万个处于芳香不定域系统中的碳原子组成的大分子，以团聚的方式存在；石墨烯材料层与层之间的范德瓦耳斯力使其容易相互聚集。因此，没有经过处理的碳纳米材料难以在水中保持分散状态，会重新聚集形成块。材料表面与其他介质的界面相容性较差，呈惰性状态，难于分散在水和常用的有机溶剂等介质中。这些缺陷大大限制了碳纳米材料的生物应用[7-11]。因此，改善碳纳米材料的亲水性及亲油性，提高材料的生物相容性，克服其在应用上的限制，在与其他材料复合后发挥其优越的性能，致力于开发生物相容性好、更能适应人体生理需要的新材料始终是碳纳米材料生物医学应用领域的研究热点[7,8]。

目前，实验室一般采用表面接枝（化学接枝、物理接枝）、等离子体技术（等离子体表面聚合、等离子体表面处理、等离子体化学气相沉积、等离子体喷涂）、离子束技术（离子束注入、离子束沉积、离子束辅助沉积）、电化学沉积技术等方式在碳纳米材料表面接入羧基、羟基、磺酸基、氨基、亚氨基、酰胺基等官能团，达到改变材料的物理和化学性质的目的。这些功能性基团可赋予碳纳米材料一些新的特性，例如分散性、亲水性、与聚合物的兼容性、促细胞生长和黏附等，从而获得生物相容性较好的碳纳米材料[12,13]。

离子束技术是在物理学、化学、电子学、真空技术等学科基础上交叉发展形成的一门新兴技术。相比于其他表面修饰方式，离子束技术具有无可替代的技术优势：① 它能在常温下进行，不会因温度因素对修饰材料产生影响；② 在真空中进行，对修饰材料无污染；③ 引入的元素可以任意选择，不受合金系统中固溶体的限制；④ 引入元素剂量可精确控制；⑤ 仅使材料表层的成分、结构发生变化，并且可通过选择修饰方式及改变能量控制注入粒子浓度-深度的分布，改变材料与生物体相互作用的特性，但不影响修饰材料的内部结构和性能，无附着等问题；⑥ 条件可控，具有可靠性和重复性[14]。因此，鉴于离子束修饰的技术优势，我们围绕碳纳米材料（碳纳米管、石墨烯），利用离子束技术进行了大量的研究工作，并取得了一些实验结果。

1. 一维碳纳米材料：多壁碳纳米管的表面修饰及生物相容性研究

碳纳米管作为一维碳纳米材料的典型代表，具有大的比表面积、超轻的质量、丰富的电子结构、良好的导电性、高的机械强度、高的化学和热稳定性等一系列独特理化性质。它一直是医学诊断、处理、治疗、各种生物传感器等领域的热门研究材料。生物相容性评价作为生物材料临床应用前的基础性评价，是应用及开发碳纳米管生物性能的必要评价手段。根据我们早期针对碳纳米管的生物相容性开展工作发现：在碳纤维上附着多壁碳纳米管（multi-walled carbon nanotube，MWCNT）能够促进细胞黏附、生长，并具有一定的抗凝血、溶血性能[15,16]。但是，在实验的过程中我们也发现了 MWCNT 的强疏水性在一定程度上起到了抑制 MWCNT 的生物相容性提高的作用。为此，我们用化学法制备的含氮多壁碳纳米管（nitrogen-doped multi-walled carbon nanotube, N-MWCNT）取代 MWCNT。尽管这种方法制备的 N-MWCNT 中氮元素是以结构组分的形式，少量的存在于竹节状结构当中，并且该材料并未达到改善 MWCNT 疏水性的目的，但生物实验仍然取得了很好的结果[16]。这说明以氮元素为代表的亲水性基团具有促生物相容性的功能；并且也提示我们采用新的修饰方法将活性基团尽可能的留在材料表面，而非参与结构，因为材料的生物相容性在很大程度上取决于材料表面的物理和化学性质。

在这种思想的指导下，我们从 3 个方面开展了工作：① 采用离子束辅助沉积（ion beam assisted deposition, IBAD）技术在 MWCNT 表面沉积纳米碳氮（$CN_x$）薄膜[17,18]；② 采用 IBAD 技术对 MWCNT 进行低能氮离子束轰击[19,20]；③ 采用离子注入（ion implantation）技术将 $NH_2^+$、$COOH^+$ 离子引入 MWCNT[21,22]。这些尝试仅改变了 MWCNT 的表层理化性质，并未引起 MWCNT 本身结构的变化。因此，不仅 MWCNT 本身的空间拓扑结构，大的比表面积、孔隙率等优势得以保留及发挥，同时借用了修饰成分本身的活性、亲水性和较好的生物相容性。实验结果表明：这 3 种修饰方法均有效地改善了 MWCNT 的亲水性，大幅度提高了细胞在修饰材料表面的黏附与生长，并达到抗凝血、溶血的性能。

另一方面，通过对比 3 组实验结果，我们也发现了 3 种方法各自的特点。① 相较于离子注入，IBAD 技术产生的轰击离子能量较低，所以传递给修饰离子的能量也较低，大量修饰离子会停留在 MWCNT 表层，而使用离子注入技术引入的修饰离子会在 MWCNT 表面一定深度范围呈现高斯分布；② IBAD 束流较大，即产生的轰击离子较多，相比离子注入技术更易大量的引入修饰粒子；③ IBAD 技术不仅能够引入离子，同时还能实现 MWCNT 表面成膜，这在提高 MWCNT 血液相容性方面具有离子注入技术无法相比的优势；④ IBAD 技术在引入修饰离子方面具有限制性，例如，含氧离子易与灯丝反应，无法使用 IBAD 技术实现，相较之下离子注入可实现的修饰离子范围更广，种类更多；⑤ 离子注入的磁过滤装置对修饰离子具有筛选性，因此，修饰离子的纯度更高，更不易产生杂质。

2. 二维碳纳米材料：石墨烯（graphene）的表面修饰及生物相容性研究

石墨烯作为二维碳纳米材料的代表，具有大的比表面积，良好的结构刚性、优良的电导率、柔韧性、表面可功能化的特性，这些特性使其在生物材料领域具有良好的应用前景。尤其是其平整的表面结构使其具有明显优于 MWCNT 的抗凝血性能。但石墨烯也同样存在疏水性强的缺陷。为了改善石墨烯的疏水性，进一步提高生物相容性，我们择优选择离子注入这一修饰方式在石墨烯表面引入 $N^+$、$NH_2^+$、$COOH^+$ 离子[23,24]，发现这些活性基团有效地提高了石墨烯的亲水性，细胞在修饰后的石墨烯表面形态扁平，伪足粗壮，增殖数量大；而血小板在修饰后的石墨烯表面则黏附数量较少，形态保持完好，几乎没有发生变形和集聚。说明 $N^+$、$NH_2^+$、$COOH^+$ 离子的引入很好地达到了改善、提高石墨烯生物相容性的效果；并且随着引入活性离子的增多，显现出更优的生物相容性。

3. 三维碳纳米材料：3D 石墨烯的表面修饰及细胞相容性研究

虽然二维石墨烯经过修饰后体现出大的比表面积，良好的结构刚性，优良的电导率、柔韧性、亲水性等优势，但也显现出其平面二维结构的缺陷：难于形成可供细胞生长与组织修复所需的三维结构。因此，制备三维石墨烯体材料，将三维石墨烯作为组织支架，为纳米材料、微米细胞、宏观组织之间搭建一座联系的桥梁[25-27]，成为我们近阶段研究工作的关注点。

我们利用离子注入技术将 $N^+$ 离子引入通过水热合成法制备的 3D 石墨烯中。原始的氧化石墨在超声分离后形成氧化石墨烯溶液，溶液在一定的水热条件下进行自组装反应，还原过程中，石墨烯片层相互堆叠，层与层之间依靠离子力和范德瓦耳斯力支撑，形成立体结构的自主装石墨烯凝胶。该凝胶体具有均匀的、微米直径的多孔状结构。经过 $N^+$ 离子注入后，3D 石墨烯的孔径尺寸和宏观整体形貌均未发生明显改变，大部分 N 以活性离子的形式存在于材料表面，一部分 N 元素与石墨烯片层上的 C 元素相结合，甚至替代了石墨烯本身的 C 元素，破坏了石墨烯本身的六角型蜂巢结构，形成碳氮掺杂、吡咯氮、吡啶氮等多种掺杂形式。且随着离子注入浓度的增加，3D 石墨烯的缺陷程度增加，含 N 官能团的含量不断增高。这些含 N 官能团在体液环境下解离，携带正电荷，这些正电荷与带负电荷的蛋白发生静电作用，增强蛋白吸附；而黏附蛋白又进一步为细胞黏附、增殖提供活性位点，有效提高了 3D 石墨烯的细胞相容性。

综上所述，最近几年我们围绕从一维到三维的碳纳米材料的离子束表面修饰及其在生物领域的应用开展了一系列研究，取得了一定成果，使得不具备生物相容性的碳材料在生物领域的应用成为可能，这为进一步在生物医学领域利用碳纳米材料的一系列优势打下基础。与此同时，我们也认识到了碳材料在生物领域应用的更深层次的问题，例如，碳材料的代谢问题。在未来的工作中我们将致力于解决这一系列问题。路漫漫其修远兮，吾将上下而求索。

# 培养期间代表性文章

1. Li D J, Cui F Z, Gu H Q. $F^+$ ion implantation induced cell attachment on intraocular lens. *Biomaterials*, 1999, 20 (20)：1889-1896.

**Abstract** Cell attachment on the polymethylmethacrylate (PMMA) intraocular lens (IOL) was studied by ion implantation. $F^+$ ion implantation was performed at an energy of 80 keV with fluences ranging from $5\times10^{12}$ to $5\times10^{15}$ ions/cm$^2$ at room temperature. The cell attachment tests gave interesting results in that the number of the platelets, the neutral granulocytes, and the macrophages adhering on the surface of the IOLs was reduced significantly after F$^+$ ion implantation. The optimal fluence was about $3\times10^{14}$ to $4\times10^{14}$ ions/cm$^2$. The hydrophobicity imparted to the surface was also monitored. At the same time, no appreciable change in the tensile strength and the optical transmittance of the implanted samples was observed. X-ray photoelectron spectroscopy (XPS) and fourier transfer infrared (FTIR) analysis showed that F$^+$ ion implantation caused the cleavage of some pendants, the oxidation of the surface, and the formation of some new F-containing groups. These results were responsible for the cell attachment changes.

引用次数：**35**

2. Li D J, Cui F Z, Gu H Q. Studies of diamond-like carbon films coated on PMMA by ion beam assisted deposition. *Applied Surface Science*, 1999, 137 (1-4): 30-37.

**Abstract**    Diamond-like carbon (DLC) films on polymethylmethacrylate (PMMA) substrates were prepared using ion beam assisted deposition. The carbon films deposited by Ar$^+$ sputtering graphite were simultaneously bombarded by CH$^{n+}$ at the bombarding energies of $200-1000$ eV. The morphology, structure, and bonding states of the films were characterized by Scanning electron microscopy, X-ray photoelectron spectroscopy, Raman spectroscopy, and UV-visible absorption spectroscopy respectively. Results showed that DLC films were amorphous and smooth with higher fraction of sp$^3$ bonds in the structure of mixed sp$^3$ + sp$^2$ bonding. The friction coefficient of the DLC/PMMA system was examined.

引用次数：**26**

# 参考文献

[1]    Kroto H W, Heath J R, Obrien S C, et al. C60: Buck minster fullerene [J]. *Nature*, 1985, 318: 162-163.

[2]    Iijima S. Helical microtubules of graphitic carbon [J]. *Nature*, 1991, 354: 56-58.

[3]    Novoselov K S, Geim A K, Morozov S V, et al. Electric field effect in atomically thin carbon films [J]. *Science*, 2004, 306: 666-669.

[4]    Peng X G. Band gap and composition engineering on a nanocrystal (BCEN) in solution [J]. *Accounts of Chemical Research*, 2010, 43: 1387-1395.

[5]    Hedenmo M, Narvaez A, Dominguez E, et al. Improved mediated tyrosinase amperometric enzyme electrode [J]. *Journal of Electroanalytical Chemistry*, 1997, 425: 1-11.

［6］　Wang J. Miniaturized DNA biosensor for detecting cryptosporidium in water samples ［J］. *Technical Completion Report*, 2000, 26: 1-11.

［7］　Stark N J. Biological evaluation of medical devices-Part 4: selection of tests for interactions with blood ［S］. *International Standard.* ISO 10993-4: 2002 （E）: 1-17.

［8］　Wettero J, Askendal A, Bengtsson T, et al. On the binding of complement to solid artificial surfaces in vitro ［J］. *Biomaterials*, 2002, 21: 981-987.

［9］　Harrison BS, Atala A. Carbon nanotube applications for tissue engineering ［J］. *Biomaterials*, 2007, 28: 344-353.

［10］　Yang M, Yang Y, Yang H, et al. Layer-by-layer self-assembled multi-layer films of carbon nanotubes and platinum nanoparticles with poly-electrolyte for the fabrication of biosensors ［J］. *Biomaterials*, 2006, 27: 246-255.

［11］　Lacerda L, Bianco A, Prato M, et al. Carbon nanotubes as nanomedicines: From toxicology to pharmacology ［J］. *Adv. Drug Deliv. Rev.*, 2006, 58: 1460-1470.

［12］　Shan C, Yang H, Han D, et al. Water-soluble graphene covalently functionalized by biocompatible poly-l-lysine ［J］. *Langmuir*, 2009, 25: 12030-12033.

［13］　Luo J, Cote L J, Tung V C, et al. Graphene oxide nanocolloids ［J］. *J. Am. Chem. Soc.*, 2010, 132: 17667-17669.

［14］　徐晓宙. 生物材料学 ［M］. 北京: 科学出版社. 2006.

［15］　袁丽. 多壁碳纳米管的生物相容性研究 ［D］. 天津: 天津师范大学, 2010.

［16］　Zhao M L, Li D J, Yuan L, et al. Differences in cytocompatibility and hemocompatibility between carbon nanotubes and nitrogen-doped carbon nanotubes ［J］. *Carbon*, 2011, 49: 3125-3133.

［17］　Zhao M L, Li D J, Gu H Q, et al. In vitro cell adhesion and hemocompatibility of carbon nanotubes with CN$_x$ coating ［J］. *Curr. Nanosci.*, 2012, 8: 451-457.

［18］　Zhao M L, Li D J, Guo M X, et al. The different N concentrations induced cytocompatibility and hemocompatibility of MWCNTs with CN$_x$ coatings ［J］. *Surface and Coatings Technology*, 2013, 229: 90-96.

［19］　Zhao M L, Cao Y, Liu X Q, et al, Effect of nitrogen atomic percentage on N$^+$-bombarded MWCNTs in cytocompatibility and hemocompatibility ［J］. *Nano Res. Lett.*, 2014, 9: 142.

［20］　Zhao M L, Liu X Q, Cao Y, et al. Superior cell adhesion and antithrombogenicity supported by N$^+$-bombarded carbon nanotubes ［J］. *Curr. Nanosci.*, 2015, 11: 135-142.

［21］　Zhang Y T, Li M S, Zhao M L, et al. Influence of polar functional groups introduced by COOH$^+$ implantation on cell growth and anticoagulation of MWCNTs ［J］. *Journal of Materials Chemistry B*, 2013, 1: 5543-5549.

［22］　Guo M X, Li D J, Zhao M L, et al. NH$_2$$^+$ implantations induced superior hemocompatibility of carbon nanotubes ［J］. *Nanoscale Research Letters*, 2013, 8: 205 （1-6）.

［23］　Guo M X, Li M S, Liu X Q, et al. N-containing functional groups induced superior cytocompatible and hemocompatible graphene by NH$_2$ ion implantation ［J］. *J. Mater. Sci.*:

*Mater. Med.*, 2013, 24: 2741-2748.

[24] Guo M X, Li D J, Zhao M L, et al. Nitrogen ion implanted graphene as thrombo-protective safer and cytoprotective alternative for biomedical applications [J]. *Carbon*, 2013, 61: 321-328.

[25] Li N, Zhang Q, Gao S, et al. Three-dimensional graphene foam as a biocompatible and conductive scaffold for neural stem cells [J]. *Scientific Reports*, 2013, 3 (1604): 1-6.

[26] Wang I N E, Robinson J T, Do G, et al. Graphite oxide nanoparticles with diameter greater than 20 nm are biocompatible with mouse embryonic stem cells and can be used in a tissue engineering system [J]. *Small*, 2014, 10: 1479-1484.

[27] Liu L, Zhai J F, Zhu C J, et al. One-pot synthesis of 3-dimensional reduced grapheme oxide-based hydrogel as support for microbe immobilization and BOD biosensor preparation [J]. *Biosensors and Bioelectronics*, 2015, 63: 483-489.

# 3.4 敢于探索科学未知领域
## ——祝贺崔福斋教授 70 寿辰

### 范昱玮

波士顿大学，美国

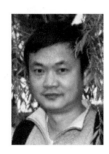

范昱玮，1998—2002 年，于清华大学材料科学与工程系攻读博士学位，师从崔福斋教授。毕业后分别在加拿大英属哥伦比亚大学和美国南加州大学从事博士后研究。后在美国新奥尔良大学担任助理研究员。现在美国波士顿大学工作。

　　回忆 18 年前和崔教授初识的那个秋季，在清华大学的工物馆，他很兴奋地给我简单指出了一个充满前景的生物材料科研领域，鼓励我报考他的博士生。作为化工材料专业的硕士生，对生物的了解仅限于高中那点零星的知识，现代的生物技术完全不懂。那个时代正是生物学科高速发展的起步时期，我怀着对未知的渴望加入了崔教授的课题组。

　　研究组不算大，三位高年级的师兄、师姐挤在工物馆小小的实验室里，但每位师兄、师姐都做不同方向的大课题，从材料抗菌机理、骨修复到仿生涂层，第一次的组会上我听得远山雾罩的，崔老师时不时给出一些简洁的评价。很快我就要开始选题，大方向是细胞与材料的相互作用，特别是中枢神经再生。我当时就觉得蒙了，中枢神经可以再生么？崔老师让我查一下文献，早点开始动手做实验。但是做什么，他没说。我查了一个多月的文献资料，就去找崔老师抱怨，这个领域基本没啥可参考的，已发表的相关文章的数量基本是个位数，我打算换一个可以开展的课题。崔教授当时很有前瞻地说："正是没有前人的研究结果，咱们才要去做，你的这个方向不仅在国内，而且在国际上也是少有人去研究的，但是研究结果意义重大。"经过这次谈话，我的兴趣被激发了很多。崔老师建议我去学生物系的课程，例如生物化学、神经生物学。那时候电子版的文献还是很稀少的，我经常跑校图书馆、北京图书馆、军事医学科学院图书馆，甚至北京大学医学部的图书馆。从 70 年代初的文献查起，看看其他人如何在体外培养神经组织或者在体内促进神经再生。同时，根据崔教授的建议，我开始和杜昶师兄学习细胞培养技术、材料表面处理，在生物系学习基础生化知识。

一年过去了，我的基础知识和技术不断积累，我见过崔老师几次，和他讨论实验的计划。经过一段时间的文献阅读，我对这个研究有了很大的兴趣，逐渐产生两个研究方向的想法：一个是建立神经元与体外通讯的界面，可以用于人机信号交流；另一个是利用水凝胶促进三维神经系统的再生。似乎就像在实现一些科幻小说或电影里再生大脑中枢系统的功能，或者建立连接人脑和计算机的通信，可以用于计算机读取神经信号。哪一个方向可以出结果，崔教授并不对我直接说明。但是他鼓励我两个都做，假如一个不成功，还有另一个保证可以完成学位论文。

但是从科学畅想回到现实，当时我们一直没有神经培养和神经生物学的技术，崔老师推荐我去找合作。杜昶师兄合作的医院的医生也没有这方面经验，我们尝试自己培养神经细胞，均未成功。我开始联系北京大学、北京协和医院、北京大学医学部的相关研究组，他们对这种课题表示感兴趣，但更多的是惊讶。直到 1999 年初，我在文献中看到首都医科大学神经科学研究所一直在做帕金森病的研究，我找到主管这个研究所的徐群渊教授，他表示出很大的兴趣并愿意合作，还介绍了一位医学博士生与我协作。于是，我开始做一些体外的神经细胞培养，主要是大鼠的黑质细胞。

1999 年初，当组织培养有了合作的时候，实验进展就容易一些了。不过，最初一两次实验确实是基本不成功的，北京大学医学部的研究人员也从来没有在培养板以外的材料上养过神经细胞，包括如何观察非透明材料上的细胞也是一个问题。在和崔老师以及北京大学医学部的同事讨论后，我们总结了一些容易出问题的操作环节，很快我们可以在经过物理和化学处理的硅片表面培养神经元细胞，并且通过荧光显微镜和扫描电子显微镜观察到细胞的结构。紧接着下一年水凝胶的研究方向也有了进展。兴奋之余，崔老师却严厉地说：如果实验结果不能发表就不是有价值的数据，让我抓紧围绕发表文章的目的去做实验。写文章和投稿对我是全新的经历，崔老师基本上是逐字逐句和我一起修改语法，研读文献，处理图标。研究组的师兄也帮忙修改文章草稿，经过不下10 轮的修改，崔老师才觉得文章基本可以投出去了。而且，那时候投稿还需要去邮局邮寄，非常慢。等了 4 个多月，审稿意见才回来，需要小的修改并回答几个评审人的问题。

很快我们开始整理第二篇文章，主要结果是有了，但我们发现黑质细胞在不同腐蚀程度的硅片表面有不同的附着程度，是由表面的化学键不同，还是晶体取向不同，或者粗糙度不同引起的？经过几个月的光谱学测试，并没有合理的结果出现，实验进度一下停滞了好几个月。正巧，实验室的原子力显微镜开始安装，很快我得到了表明粗糙度的数据，并通过光刻蚀法制作了具有不同粗糙度的微图案的硅片，很快细胞培养结果也表明黑质细胞确实有选择性地附着在不同粗糙度表面上。同时，水凝胶组织工程的课题实验也顺利进入动物实验阶段。在课题进行中，思维很快就开阔了，有很多其他的想法去做。期间，崔老师一直提醒我要注意，发表好文章是科研的主要目的，不要为了一些小的兴趣偏离了主题。只有完备的实验结果被发表了，才能说明是被大家承认的好的科研。

我在读博士期间在 SCI 收录期刊上一共发表了 4 篇文章，在中文期刊上合作发表了 5 篇文章，申请到 1 项中国专利。其中关于不同粗糙度表面对神经细胞的影响发表在神经生物学的期刊 *Journal of Neuroscience Methods* 上，到 2015年的 SCI 引用超过了 135 次，而且有大量的近期引用，足以显示在十几年前崔老师帮助我选题和设计实验的前瞻性。有些文章认为我们是最早进行有关纳米尺度材料和神经细胞相互作用的研究。美国在 2014 年开始投入新的一轮对大脑结构和功能的深入研究，主要的一个手段是利用大视场扫描电子显微镜对脑结构做纳米尺度的测绘，目的还是神经再生和功能重建。毕业后很遗憾没有继续在同一方向进行科研，但是我还继续在生物材料领域做科研和教学。在清华大学生物材料研究组，大家经常进行学术讨论，学术气氛高涨，所以我对各种课题方向都有一些了解，这也奠定了我后来能够在不同学科交叉课题进行科研的基础。崔老师对我科研能力的培养是具有长期影响的，特别是独立科研能力和协作能力，在清华大学做的几个研究方向都是在几乎没有前人参照的基础上开始的，这对科研工作者的源动力是极大的锻炼。

在崔老师 70 寿辰之际，回忆一下当年在清华大学和导师一起追逐科研梦想的日子，祝愿他老人家身体康健，也祝愿生物材料研究组发展壮大。

## 培养期间代表性文章

1. Fan Y W, Cui F Z, Hou S P, Xu Q Y, Chen L N, Lee I S. Culture of neural cells on silicon wafers with nano-scale surface topograph. *Journal of Neuroscience Methods*, 2002, 120（1）: 17-23.

**Abstract** The adherence and viability of central neural cells（substantia nigra）on a thin layer of $SiO_2$ on Si wafers with different surface roughness were investigated. Variable roughness of the Si wafer surface was achieved by etching. The nano-scale surface topography was evaluated by atomic force microscopy. The adherence and subsequent viability of the cells on the wafer were examined by scanning electron microscopy（SEM）and fluorescence immunostaining of tyrosine hydroxylase (TH) . It is found that the surface roughness significantly affected cell adhesion and viability. Cells survived for over 5 days with normal morphology and expressed neuronal TH when grown on surfaces with an average roughness (Ra) ranging from 20 to 50 nm. However, cell adherence was adversely affected when surfaces with Ra less than 10 nm and rough surfaces with Ra above 70 nm were used as the substrate. Such a simple preparation procedure may provide a suitable interface surface for silicon-based devices and neurones or other living tissues.

引用次数：**142**

2. Fan Y W, Cui F Z, Chen L N, Zhai Y, Xu Q Y, Lee I S. Adhesion of neural cells on silicon wafer with nano-topographic surface. *Applied Surface Science*, 2002, 187 (3-4): 313-318.

**Abstract**　The adherence and subsequent viability of central neural cells (substantia nigra) on silicon wafers with different surface roughness conditions were investigated. Various roughness conditions of the silicon wafer were achieved by etching at different times. The topography was evaluated by AFM. Primary neurons were obtained from Wistar rats. The adherence and subsequent viability of the cells on the wafer were examined by scanning electronic microscopy and fluorescence immunostaining of tyrosine hydroxylase. It is found that the surface roughness affects significantly cell adhesion and viability. Cells can survive for over 5 days on the surface with average roughness in the range 20−70 nm. Such a treatment may provide a new method to make a mild interface of silicon-based electronic devices and neurons as well as other living tissues.

引用次数：**34**

# 3.5 献给崔福斋教授 70 周岁生日

## 张 伟

国家纳米科学中心，北京

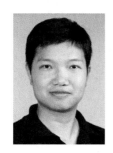

张伟，分别于 1999 年和 2004 年在清华大学材料科学与工程系获学士学位和博士学位，博士导师为崔福斋教授，博士期间主要从事生物矿化机理及骨修复材料的研究，毕业论文题目为《胶原/磷酸钙生物矿化机理研究》。2004—2006 年，在美国纽约州立大学布法罗分校化学系从事博士后研究工作；2006—2008 年，在深圳清华大学研究院从事研究工作；2008 年 7 月，被聘为国家纳米科学中心副研究员；2014 年 3 月至今被聘为国家纳米科学中心研究员。当前主要围绕组织工程中材料与细胞相互作用的基本问题，以微纳米技术和表面化学为手段，开发可以用于组织工程的新材料，为组织工程研究提供了新思路。主要科研工作包括：利用生物材料和微纳米结构技术构建体外组织结构；基于表面化学和微纳米结构的细胞生物学研究方法的建立及相关研究；材料的表面修饰、功能化研究及应用等。在 *Adv. Mater.*、*Adv. Funct. Mater.*、*Small*、*Angew. Chem. Int. Ed.*、*Lab Chip*、*Anal. Chem.*、*Langmuir* 等国内外学术期刊上共发表文章 53 篇，共被引用 1 000 余次。已申请发明专利 27 项，已授权 7 项。

　　青年人多梦想，常为人所鼓励。能否梦想成真，决定于两个因素：一是自己的努力，二是客观所赋予的机遇。1999 年 9 月，满怀对研究生生活的期待及对科研生活的憧憬，我进入了崔福斋教授的研究组开始了我的科学人生。

　　科学在现代社会生活中起中心作用，科学与人生也是密不可分得。科学人生起源于对科学的好奇，发现然后提出问题，进而探索科学的秘密。科学奠基人贝尔纳（Bernard）强调："课题的形成和选择，无论作为外部的经济要求，抑或作为科学本身的要求，都是研究工作中最复杂的一个阶段。一般来说，提出课题比解决课题更困难。……所以评价和选择课题，便成了研究的起点。"进入研究组后，在崔福斋教授的指导下，在研究组师兄、师姐的帮助下，刚走进实验室的我开始阅读研究组相关研究领域里最近的权威综述文献，经过一段时间的阅读后，会定期与崔老师交流讨论，接受崔老师的点评。崔老师对课题的把握、对学科领域的学科视野、丰富的研究经验等都对我产生了重要影响。在崔老师的指导下，我的阅读变得更有效、更省力。在崔老师的帮助下，一步一步地搞清楚我所感兴趣的研究领域里已解决的和未解决的问题。最后，从这些综述中选出几个我感兴趣的，在这领域里已被公认的、接受的概念和假说。并且最终确定了我的研究题目为《胶原/磷酸钙生物矿化机理研究》。该研究工作的主要创新性来源于学科交叉，我的研究工作是生物矿化，但是与化学上的自组装结合，最终产生了创新的认识。现代自然科学重大的理论突破和理论问题的解决，大多是科学交叉的产物。重大新技术的出现，不再只是来源于单纯经验性的创造发明，它更经常地来源于科学研究的交叉。当时生物矿化研究的主要目标是理解有机物参与的控制过程，以及生物矿化与无机矿化的差别。但是大部分的研究主要集中在有机分子控制下无机晶体的成核和生长，几乎没有研究关注矿化过程中的有机分子的状态。为了弄清楚这个问题，我们设计了相关实验，做了多次尝试。在科研实践过程中，崔老师教会我们的不只是如何解决实验中遇到的问题，更培养了我们分析问题、解决问题的能力。通过不断的努力，最终我们获得了胶原矿化过程中构象改变的实验证据：我们通过圆二色谱实时监测胶原矿化过程中胶原的二级构象，显示出胶原构象的改变。通过紫外分光光度计研究胶原/磷酸钙体外矿化体系，在浊度监测中采用更短的采样间隔首次发现初始矿化中存在一个凝胶化过程。激光光散射强度随反应时间的变化也遵循与浊度变化相同的规律。在凝胶化点，胶原构象迅速改变，同时无定形的磷酸钙相变成结晶很好的 $CaHPO_4 \cdot 2H_2O$。凝胶化现象在生物体内的矿化过程中都普遍存在，因此，胶原/磷酸钙凝胶化机理的研究，对研究人体内的自然生物矿化机理有十分重要的意义。

生物矿化是围绕生物矿物的形成过程和机制的阐明而发展起来的科学。生物矿物最早是在 20 世纪矿物学家研究活组织形成的矿物时命名的，这些生物矿物有化石、贝壳等。后来因为这个研究对象涉及有机物质，特别是与生物矿物有关的生物分子，例如蛋白质、细胞、DNA，所以生物矿化研究人员逐渐从矿物学家、地质学家扩大范围到有机化学家、生物学家等。近年来，随着有机物调制无机晶体成核长大以及其中相互作用的机制研究的深入，材料科学家、医药学家和仿生工程专家也加入到生物矿化研究之中，并应用其中的原理探索更重要的应用，例如矿化胶原的骨移植材料、纳米自组装功能材料等。新型骨、牙修复材料以及其他先进工程材料的仿生制备依赖于矿化胶原纤维结构研究的进一步发展。我们试图理解关于胶原矿化的一些基本科学问题，包括天然骨的矿化胶原纤维组成、微观结构、晶体学特征以及有机-无机相之间的关系等。

骨和牙本质是具有高度复杂分级结构的矿化胶原材料，我们按照仿生的思路设计和制备了矿化胶原纳米纤维的分级自组装并深入研究了矿化胶原纤维结构的组装机制。发现胶原纤维调制纳米羟基磷灰石晶体在其表面沉积，并具有与天然矿化相同的择优取向，多根矿化胶原纤维平行排列组成胶原纤维簇。研究结果发表在 *Chemistry of Materials* 上，文章被材料领域权威期刊 *Nature Materials* 作为 Research Notes 专文评述（Synthetic bone，*Nature Materials*，2003，2 (9)：566-566），给予了很高的评价，认为我们的研究工作"给出第一个直接的体外证据，证明了相关的矿化理论……将提高人类对其他各种矿化组织中胶原调制矿化机理的理解，并为仿生工程制备新型功能材料指明道路"（giving the first direct evidence to support previous theories that this occurs. …These results should improve the understanding of collagen-mediated mineralization in other calcified tissues，and point the way to new functional materials for biomimetic engineering）。美国化学学会主页专文发表评论，认为是发现了人骨中矿化胶原纤维自组装的"关键机理"（They have found a key mechanism behind how these fibrils self-assemble）。另外，在化学领域的权威综述期刊 *Chemical Review* 第 108 卷，第 11 期上，由著名材料学家、美国西北大学教授 Samuel I. Stupp 等人撰写的综述文章 *Biomimetic systems for hydroxyapatite mineralization inspired by bone and enamel* 中，不仅引用了我们发表的矿化胶原纳米纤维多级组装的电镜照片，而且大段引用我们的论述，肯定了我们的实验结果（More recently，Zhang et al. attempted to replicate the hierarchical self-assembly of mineralized collagen into composites of nanofibrils. HA crystals grew on the surface of triple helical fibrils such that their c-axes were oriented along the long axis of the fibrils，as in natural bone. The hierarchical structure of the composite was verified by conventional and high-resolution TEM）。

生物矿化过程对生物进化和生态环境有很多重要的启示。从纳米级别的蛋白世界、某些细菌中的磁性指南针到介观尺度的牡蛎壳、珊瑚、象牙、骨骼和牙釉质，生物体发展了一套系统的化学体系，将硬物质和软物质结合起来，设计合成具有各种功能性的有机无机复合材料。这些启示从空间尺度上可以说是全球范围的，从时间尺度上可以追溯到生命的起源。所以，生物矿化研究是一个从古生物学、海洋化学、沉积学、医学和牙科学中分离出来的交叉学科，它强调在化学、生物学和材料科学的多学科交叉中开展工作。未来的前沿科研工作也会出现在多学科交叉融合之处，例如可穿戴设备，首先是与人体关系紧密的基础医疗器械，同时上面集成微电路、微探测器、微处理器等，为提高信号检测和处理传输性能，还可以进一步结合表面纳米技术、微流控技术等。在生物进化中，大自然已经给我们呈现了各式各样的奇特的无机结构。每一个物种合成了各种带有它们物种特色的生物矿物。这些生物矿化过程是由生物从基因到蛋白再到物理化学分子水平控制的。随着生物化学和分子生物学以及材料科学的发展，从分子水平解析生物矿化机制成为可能。生物矿化的基本原理和分子机制也将为我们进行生物硬组织（骨骼、牙齿）修复和病理性矿化的预防治疗提供思路和方法。此外，生物矿化过程机理为制备具有特殊功能的仿生材料提供了新的思路。"仿生设计"作为一种研究方法在各个领域都为科学家们所重视和利用，例如，早期飞机的结构就是模仿鸟类和昆虫，红外线探测器的研究是受到了响尾蛇的启发，声呐的出现则是受到海豚本能的启示。生物矿化领域的未来发展也不例外，生物矿化中的自组装、反馈和模拟将为合成生物活性陶瓷、功能生物材料等领域提供新的理论。仿生矿化研究是仿生材料研究的一个重点分支方向。仿生矿化以研究生物体中的矿物质为基础，目的是在对生物矿物材料的了解基础上模仿生物体，合成具有相似结构和性能的矿物材料，例如碳酸钙、羟基磷灰石等，这些材料结构和功能的创建在建筑和人造骨骼等方面有着广阔的应用前景。自然通过优胜劣汰选择继承和发展下来的生物体十分复杂，其自身合成的特殊材料及其"神奇"的性质和功能不禁让人们对大自然的鬼斧神工惊叹不已。针对这些微观材料和结构的模仿将是未来仿生材料合成的重点和难点方向。目前，仿生材料的研究还有很长的路要走。对生物体自身材料的原理和合成方法还需要进一步的探索。各种合成影响因素也需进一步研究。模拟自然材料仅仅是第一步，重在创新，更主要的是从理念上把握材料合成的精髓，找出经济、方便的合成路径，创造性地将仿生材料运用到人类的实际生活中去，从而真正起到造福人类的作用。

# 培养期间代表性文章

1. Zhang W, Liao S S, Cui F Z. Hierarchical self-assembly of nano-fibrils in mineralized collagen. *Chemistry of Materials*, 2003, 15 (16): 3221-3226.

**Abstract**  A designed hierarchical structure was made by self-assembly of nano-fibrils of mineralized collagen resembling extracellular matrix. The collagen fibrils were formed by self-assembly of collagen triple helices. Hydroxyapatite (HA) crystals grew on the surface of these fibrils in such a way that their c-axes were oriented along the longitudinal axes of the fibrils. The mineralized collagen fibrils aligned parallel to each other to form mineralized collagen fibers. For the first time, the new hierarchical self-assembly structure of collagen-hydroxyapatite composite was verified by conventional and high-resolution transmission electron microscopy.

引用次数：**244**

2. Zhang W, Huang Z L, Liao S S, Cui F Z. Nucleation sites of calcium phosphate crystals during collagen mineralization. *Journal of the American Ceramic Society*, 2003, 86 (6): 1052-1054.

**Abstract**    The nucleation sites of calcium phosphate crystals during collagen mineralization were studied by Fourier transform infrared spectrometry and transmission electron microscopy. It was found for the first time that there is another nucleation site, i. e. , carbonyl ($>C=O$) on collagen, besides the previous reported nucleation site of carboxyl ($-COOH$) . By comparing the IR spectra of collagen not only with collagen/calcium phosphate but also with collagen/$Ca^{2+}$, it was observed that the peak intensities of amides I , II , and III of collagen decreased significantly after mineralization. The decrease of the amide I peak intensity was mainly due to blockage of the $C=O$ stretch. Furthermore, the peak for amide I gradually shifted to a lower wavenumber during collagen mineralization. This shift indicated that chemical interaction between carboxyl groups and $Ca^{2+}$ ions formed in the mineralizaton.

引用次数: **65**

# 3.6 仿生骨修复材料的研发
## ——同步于骨组织工程研究和相应的医疗器械应用开发

### 廖素三

南洋理工大学，新加坡

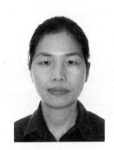

廖素三，在清华大学获博士学位后，在日本北海道大学从事两年博士后研究，接着在新加坡南洋理工大学从事博士后研究，现为新加坡南洋理工大学副教授。一直从事生物材料的研发工作。

　　2000—2003 年，在清华大学崔老师的研究组里读博士期间是人生中最充实的阶段：快速地吸收消化新知识，制定实验方案，熬夜做实验，与医生们合作学习动物实验，与企业合作申请产品临床试验许可。

　　首先，我的研究课题是《骨组织工程仿生材料的研究》，我对这个题目非常感兴趣。作为非生物材料背景的学生，每天接触的医学和生物相关知识都深深吸引和激励我更加主动深入地学习。组里师兄、师姐们前期做的天然骨结构的基础研究工作也为仿生材料的构思提供了强大的依据。同时，结合组织工程的新概念，考虑骨修复的临床应用和未来产品化的可能。组织工程本来就是跨学科的研究领域，需要考虑医疗需求、细胞反应、材料支架以及生长因子的共同作用。骨组织工程作为先于其他复杂器官和组织的研究，主要也是得益于天然骨本身结构、成分、性能的深入研究和各种骨细胞的功能及相互影响。组里一直以来做了不少天然骨结构的基础研究。跨学科的研究课题是现在做研究的常态，不局限于某一个单一领域，刚开始可能会觉得很困难，不过很有可能碰撞出许多新的想法。

　　我博士论文中首选的支架材料是以胶原/纳米羟基磷灰石为主的可降解材

料。选的细胞是成骨细胞，当然，随着干细胞研究的发展，现在更多的是用干细胞或干细胞分化的成骨细胞。选的生长因子是 BMP（bone morphogenetic protein）。分级仿生的骨组织工程材料（培养期间代表性文章 1）结合细胞实验和动物实验的结果，发表于美国生物材料学会的期刊。深入的细胞实验和三维细胞培养（培养期间代表性文章 2）的结果也发表在生物高分子材料相关期刊。对骨材料的体外和体内降解行为的研究结果（培养期间代表性文章 3）发表于 *Tissue Engineering* 上。骨材料植入脊椎的动物实验结果（培养期间代表性文章 4）发表于 *Journal of Bioactive and Compatible Polymers* 上。组织工程的发展也是随着生物材料、生物技术及细胞生物学等的发展而取得的飞跃式的进步。现在许多组织工程概念已经用于临床试验。有的生物材料结合干细胞也开始在临床领域试验。尤其对许多重大疾病，例如器官移植、心血管疾病，甚至癌症的研究都与组织工程结合起来寻找有效的研究模型和治疗的措施。

研究的生物材料是否能用于临床而且进一步产品化呢？即使材料表征、细胞实验和动物实验的结果都很好，也还需要进行全面的生物安全性评价。骨科植入是属于长期植入的第三类医疗器械，在众多医疗器械中是要求最高的一类。国外和国内都有相关的标准和条例规范，而且在不断地更新、发展和完善。那时候是第一次了解 GMP（Good Manufacturing Practice）和 ISO 10993，了解到医疗器械生产的严格要求，具体还和实际生产流程和干净的生产环境等有关因素结合起来。医疗器械的发展大大提高了整个医疗系统的有效性，病人和医生相应地有更多的选择。但是，严格的医疗器械审批管理系统也是保护病人不可缺少的。最近，我和同事们还撰写了医疗器械标准规范相关的书，其中有具体细节供参考，包括 GCP（Good Clinical Practice），这里就不多写了。非常欣喜地看到经过多年的临床试验证明安全有效的仿生骨材料拿到美国 FDA 的 510（K）的批准，成功进入美国市场。

# 培养期间代表性文章

1. Liao S S, Cui F Z, Zhang W, Feng Q L. Hierarchically biomimetic bone scaffold materials：Nano-HA/collagen/PLA composite. *Journal of Biomedical Materials Research Part B：Applied Biomaterials*，2004，69B（2）：158-165.

**Abstract**　A bone scaffold material（nano-HA/collagen/PLA composite）was developed by biomimetic synthesis. It shows some features of natural bone both in main composition and hierarchical microstructure. Nano-hydroxyapatite and collagen assembled into mineralized fibril. The three-dimensional porous scaffold materials mimic the microstructure of cancellous bone. Cell culture and animal model tests showed that the composite material is bioactive. The osteoblasts were separated from the neonatal rat calvaria. Osteoblasts adhered, spread, and proliferated throughout the pores of the scaffold material within a week. A 15-mm segmental defect model in the radius of the rabbit was used to evaluate the bone-remodeling ability of the composite. Combined with 0.5 mg rhBMP-2, the material block was implanted into the defect. The segmental defect was integrated 12 weeks after surgery, and the implanted composite was partially substituted by new bone tissue. This scaffold composite has promise for the clinical repair of large bony defects according to the principles of bone tissue engineering.

引用次数: **260**

2. Liao S S, Wang W, Uo M, Ohkawa S, Akasaka T, Tamura K, Cui F Z, Watari F. A three-layered nano-carbonated hydroxyapatite/collagen/PLGA composite membrane for guided tissue regeneration. *Biomaterials*, 2005, 26 (36): 7564-7571.

**Abstract**　Functional graded materials (FGM) provided us one new concept for guided tissue regeneration (GTR) membrane design with graded component and graded structure where one face of the membrane is porous thereby allowing cell growth thereon and the opposite face of the membrane is smooth, thereby inhibiting cell adhesion in periodontal therapy. The goal of the present study was to develop a three-layered graded membrane, with one face of 8% nano-carbonated hydroxyapatite/collagen/poly (lactic-co-glycolic acid) (nCHAC/PLGA) porous membrane, the opposite face of pure PLGA non-porous membrane, the middle layer of 4% nCHAC/ PLGA as the transition through layer-by-layer casting method. Then the three layers were combined well with each other with flexibility and enough high mechanical strength as membrane because the three layers all contained PLGA polymer that can be easily used for practical medical application. This high biocompatibility and osteoconductivity of this biodegraded composite membrane was enhanced by the nCHAC addition, for the same component and nano-level crystal size with natural bone tissue. The osteoblastic MC3T3-E1 cells were cultured on the three-layered composite membrane, the primary result shows the positive response compared with pure PLGA membrane.

引用次数: **103**

3. Liao S S, Cui F Z. In vitro and in vivo degradation of mineralized collagen-based composite scaffold: Nanohydroxyapatite/collagen/poly (L-lactide). *Tissue Engineering*, 2004, 10 (1-2): 73-80.

**Abstract**　The objective of this article was to investigate the in vitro and in vivo biodegradation of a novel biomimetic bone scaffold composite, nanohydroxyapatite/

collagen/poly（L-lactide）, that could be used for bone tissue engineering. For evaluation of in vitro degradation specimens were immersed into 1% trypsin/phosphate-buffered saline solution at 37 ℃. In vivo evaluation involved the implantation of samples into the posterolateral lumbar spine of rabbits, and the retrieved specimens were analyzed by Fourier transform-infrared spectroscopy. The results demonstrated that weight loss increased continuously in vitro with a reduction in mass of 19.6% after 4 weeks. During the experimental period in vitro, the relative rate of reduction of the three components in this material was shown to differ greatly: collagen decreased the fastest, from 40% by weight to 20% in the composite; hydroxyapatite content increased from 45 to 60%; and PLA changed little. The pore structure was maintained throughout the whole experimental period in vitro; however, the thickness of the walls of the pores decreased and the surface of the walls increased in roughness. In vivo, the ratio of collagen to hydroxyapatite appeared to be slightly higher near the transverse process than in the central part of the intertransverse process. This finding may have been due to new bone matrix formation extending from the transverse to the intertransverse process.

引用次数: **75**

4. Liao S S, Cui F Z, Zhu Y. Osteoblasts adherence and migration through three-dimensional porous mineralized collagen based composite: nHAC/PLA. *Journal of Bioactive and Compatible Polymers*, 2004, 19（2）: 117-130.

**Abstract**　Osteoblast cells were separated from the neonatal rat calvaria and co-cultured on a novel mineralized hydroxyapatite/collagen/poly（lactic acid）composite scaffold. By using this static cell culture, a three-dimensional osteoblasts/composite bone-like was constructed in vitro. The culture process was observed by scanning electron microscopy, fluorescence microscopy, confocal laser scanning microscopy, and histological analysis. Cells were observed to spread and proliferate throughout the inner-pores of the scaffold material. After a 12-day culture, the cells had grown into the interior scaffold about 200-400 μm depth of the composite by histological section observation. This mobile behavior of osteoblasts appeared to be similar to the composition and hierarchical structure of bone tissue. The adherence and migration of osteoblast cells in this three-dimensional composite is clinically important for large bone defect repair based on tissue engineering.

引用次数: **80**

# 3.7 师从自然：天然生物矿化机理研究

王秀梅

清华大学材料学院，北京

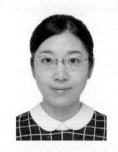

王秀梅，2005 年，于清华大学获得博士学位后，赴美国罗切斯特大学医学院和麻省理工学院生物医学工程中心从事博士后研究。自 2008 年在清华大学材料学院工作至今。生物材料方向教授，博士生导师。曾荣获 2011 年国家自然科学奖二等奖；2010—2011 年度中华医学科技奖三等奖；2014 年山东省科技进步一等奖；2012 年清华大学"学术新人奖"；入选教育部 2013 年度"新世纪优秀人才支持计划"和第 12 届霍英东教育基金会高等院校青年教师基金。

自然界是最神奇的材料设计师，也是最好的材料加工厂，在亿万年漫长的进化和演变过程中创造了不计其数光怪陆离的天然生物材料，具有独特的分级组装结构和与之完美匹配的优异性能。

天然生物矿化材料就是这样一类在自然界广泛存在的有机/无机杂化材料，例如骨骼、牙齿、珍珠、贝壳、硅藻等。尽管天然生物矿化材料种类繁多，其组成的有机、无机成分也不尽相同，但他们都有一个共同的特点，即以有机大分子调制无机矿物沉积，自组装形成复杂且高度有序的分级结构，进而实现从纳米尺度到宏观尺度的精确控制和装配。可见，由于有生命参与并控制形成过程，天然生物矿化材料具有人工合成材料无法比拟的特殊高级结构、组装方式和独特且近乎完美的性能。正是这些独特的性能引起了科学家们的兴趣，研究天然生物矿化材料形成的奥妙，揭示其高度控制机理，将为材料科学相似的控制问题提供思路，并为人工合成材料提供新的理论指导和设计依据。因此，生物矿化机理研究及其仿生模拟一直以来受到来自化学、材料、生物、考古等多个学科领域科学家们的广泛关注，同时也是中国生物材料早期研究的重点方向之一。我本人非常有幸在 2000—2005 年攻读博士学位期间一直跟随崔福斋教授从事相关领域的研究工作。

我第一次进入清华大学生物材料实验室是在 1999 年暑假。当时，大三学年刚刚结束，身边的同学都纷纷选择实验室，为读研做准备。我对生物材料这一交叉学科领域很感兴趣，虽然对其研究内涵知之甚少。在和崔老师第一次深入交谈后，更坚定了我从事生物材料研究的决心。大四学年刚刚开学，我就正式加入了崔老师的研究组，参与张漾师姐的斑马鱼脊椎骨生物矿化机理研究的课题，这也是我研究生期间一直延续的博士研究课题。我很庆幸在进实验室之初就明确了课题方向，并且坚持了下来。当时，天然生物矿化机理研究的重点主要是天然矿化材料的成分、结构分析，以及有机模板对无机晶体的调制机制的研究。但同时，人们也发现生物矿化过程本质上是受基因、蛋白、基质和细胞等逐级调制的复杂分级过程。因此，崔老师提出了从基因水平上研究生物矿化机理，探索基因如何影响蛋白编码，进而影响有机基质和后续矿化过程，这对诸如骨形成缺陷等遗传性骨疾病的理解和治疗具有重要的指导意义。我们选择斑马鱼作为生物矿化研究的模型动物，是源于一次偶然的机会了解到德国马普生物发育研究所基因生物学家 Christian Nusslein Volhard 团队的工作。他们采用化学诱变剂诱导斑马鱼基因突变，并对其进行了大规模突变体筛选，在得到的 894 个突变体中有 4 种具有成年体形畸变。我们得到对方无偿提供的这 4 种基因突变斑马鱼样本，随后开始研究这些由基因突变造成骨骼畸形的斑马鱼脊椎骨的矿化过程。斑马鱼一直以来都是发育生物学研究的最佳脊椎动物模型，我们首次将斑马鱼作为生物矿化研究模型，研究生物矿化机理。研究发现，斑马鱼脊椎骨具有和人骨非常类似的分级组装结构，我们也首次给出了斑马鱼骨分级结构模型。而基因突变后，胶原分子及其组装发生变化，引起矿化过程、分级组装结构以及力学性能的改变。尽管我们尝试通过基因测序找到影响矿化的基因突变的精确位点，但因为难度和工作量巨大而未能完成。崔老师在十几年前就提出从基因水平上研究生物矿化机理，可见其卓越的创新性、前瞻性思维和科研敏感度。

在读博的 5 年时间里，崔老师从科研选题、实验设计、成果发表等多方面给予我系统的指导，这对我后来从事科学研究影响深远。如何进行科研选题是崔老师给我讲授的第一课。科研选题重在创新，不仅要求是前人没有做过的，而且要有重要的科学价值和研究意义。所以要勇于突破常规，越是认为不可能的事情，创新性可能会越大。当然，有些奇思妙想也可能是不切实际的幻想，这就要求在选题时对前人研究基础有深入的了解。崔老师当时要求我必须阅读生物矿化领域近 10 年发表的文章。所以，从大四毕业设计开始，我就养成了阅读文献、整理文献的习惯。2000 年左右，国内的科研条件才刚刚开始有所改善。科技论文几乎没有电子版，都要到图书馆查找、复印。当时我经常跑到国家图书馆、中国科学院文献情报中心、北京协和医学院图书馆查找、复印文献和英文著作，然后再把论文分类整理、装订成册。这些资料后来留给了师弟、师妹，对他们同样很有益处。而我本人也在大量文献阅读过程中对研究课题的国际前沿动态有了更多的了解。除此之外，科学研究中一定要建立广泛合作。崔老师在科研中一直保持着开放的态度，强调合作。崔老师常常对我们说，一定要多合作，我们做生物材料研究必须要与临床医生合作，因为临床医生能够提出问题。所以，当时我们和中国人民解放军总医院、北京大学第三医院建立了长期的合作关系。在涉及斑马鱼饲养、基因分析的研究工作中，我们也和清华大学生命科学学院、军事医学科学院、首都医科大学、华大基因等实验室合作。在合作中，不同学科思维的碰撞，不仅让我的知识面逐渐拓宽，也解决了很多我在科研中的困惑。除此之外，科研成果的发表也是科研中的重要环节。崔老师常常和我们强调文章发表的重要性，科研工作做得再好，发表不出来都等于零。崔老师和我们回忆他的博士导师李恒德院士对他说的话：科学研究就像母鸡下蛋，不仅要会下蛋，还要会咯咯哒。形象的比喻让我们立刻懂得了成果发表的重要性。我的第一篇文章是在刚上博士二年级时开始撰写的。当把初稿拿给崔老师看的时候，崔老师把文章框架进行了颠覆性的修改，这也让我慢慢懂得了科技论文的写作思路和构架。随后，崔老师又进行多次细节修改，包括图片、语言、题目等。文章在寒假前投到了 *Biomaterials* 期刊上，一个月后就接收发表。当时的幸福感至今还记得。在我的第一篇科技论文撰写过程中，崔老师给予的细致指导让我至今都受益匪浅。

在我的学术生涯中，崔老师给予我的指导和帮助远不止博士期间的论文指导。我博士毕业后到美国从事博士后研究期间，也经常和崔老师交流科研上的想法。特别是在我的职业选择上，是否要继续从事科研工作，崔老师给予了我巨大的鼓励和信心。2007 年，在美国芝加哥参加 TERMIS 会议期间，见到了崔老师。我表达了回国的想法，崔老师非常支持，并鼓励我回到清华大学，继续生物材料的研究。2008 年 1 月回国后，我重新回到了清华大学生物材料研究组，没有任何陌生感，很快适应了新的工作环境。转眼回国已经 7 年了，崔老师就像我的父亲一样，见证了我在工作以及家庭生活中的每一点进步和成长。而我知道，我的每一点进步都凝聚了崔老师巨大的心血和期望，我的每一点成绩都离不开崔老师无私的帮助和支持。崔老师作为中国生物材料最早的一辈科学家，为中国生物材料的发展做出了巨大的贡献。今年，崔老师已届古稀之年，仍然工作在科研第一线，永远是我辈努力之方向。

值此崔老师 70 周岁寿辰之际，祝愿崔老师永远身体健康，开心顺意！

## 培养期间代表性文章

Wang X M, Cui F Z, Ge J, Zhang Y, Ma C. Variation of nanomechanical properties of bone by gene mutation in the zebrafish. *Biomaterials*，2002，23

(23): 4557-4563.

**Abstract**  Significant variations of nanomechanical properties and fracture morphology between gene-mutated *liliput*$^{dtc232}$ (*lilllil*) zebrafish skeletal bone and wild-type bone have been observed. Nanoindentation measurement disclosed that *lilllil* bone has 36% lower nanohardness and 32% lower elastic modulus. The standard deviations of hardness and elastic modulus of *lilllil* bone were both much higher than those of wild-type bone. SEM morphology of fracture surfaces further revealed that in bones after gene mutation, formative microcracks make the performance reduction and the increasing of brittleness. What is more, the plywood-like structure of the normal bone does not exist in the *lilllil* bone.

引用次数: **25**

# 3.8 神经修复材料的选题经历

田维明

哈尔滨工业大学生物医学工程中心，哈尔滨

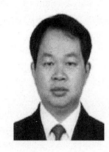
田维明，清华大学 2001 级博士研究生，博士期间主要研究透明质酸水凝胶用于中枢神经系统修复。毕业后在美国耶鲁大学医学院从事博士后研究，2009 年回国，在哈尔滨工业大学生物医学工程中心工作。目前担任生物医学工程中心副主任，教授，博士生导师。主要研究方向是生物活性水凝胶在肿瘤治疗、心肌梗死修复和干细胞调控等。

2005 年，我博士毕业离开了清华园。在崔老师的研究组里度过了难忘的博士生活，在生物材料组的点点滴滴，时常浮现在我的脑海里，回想当年的青葱岁月，恍如昨日一般。恰逢崔老师 70 寿辰，愿写一下当年选题的经历。如今我也指导着十几名研究生，看着他们选题时遇到的困难，一如我当年一般。我个人的博士选题，颇费了一番周折，我想，写出来或许对后来的师弟、师妹以及自己指导的学生有所裨益、有所启发。因此，尽管自己的文笔粗陋，还是答应把自己当年的经历呈现给大家。

2001 年的秋天，我怀揣着满心的期望和兴奋走进了清华园，进入崔老师的研究组，开始了 4 年的博士生涯。当时，对于博士课题的工作基本上没有概念，只是觉得很新奇。记得一天中午，崔老师让我和孔祥东去他家里吃饭，师母不在家，崔老师从食堂带回几个菜，又亲自下厨给我俩做了一道红烧虾，望着桌上的美食，我正想解解馋，崔老师问我们课题方向怎么想的，我俩好像都没有准备，答不上来。崔老师很严肃地给我们俩讲了毕业的要求及课题选择的重要性。我一下子紧张起来，匆匆吃了一些，都没有吃出虾的滋味。自那次从崔老师家里出来以后，就想着课题该做什么方向。刚开始的一年里，由于当时组里骨材料的研究正处于文章发表的高峰期，崔老师主要让我围绕骨修复材料进行调研，现在还清晰地记得是关于生物材料缓释质粒进行局部基因转染的研究。

一年级结束的时候，综述报告写得差不多了，正准备围绕这个方向进行实验，恰逢范煜玮大师兄毕业，他做的神经修复的材料没有人继续，崔老师就让我接着这个方向做。由于已经准备了一年的骨材料方向，并且对于脑修复材料几乎闻所未闻，心里老大不情愿，但是师命难违，就硬着头皮改换了方向。范煜玮大师兄出身高分子材料专业，对有机合成十分精通，他在研究一种高分子材料用于脑损伤修复。由于我本人对于有机合成几乎一窍不通，大师兄手把手地教我，从最基本的烧瓶清洗开始，到有机合成的关键步骤，事无巨细，无奈我化学知识十分有限，时常出错。记得当时合成的物质在最后一步要放在冰箱里过夜，第二天早上，如果看到烧瓶里有结晶沉淀，那就是我们需要的物质。当自己操作的时候，经常一无所获，自己还不知道问题出在哪里。每天早上到实验室的第一件事情就是看看有多少结晶，在开冰箱门的那一刻总是默默祷告，让我多获得一点产物吧。现在想起来还十分有趣。后来，范煜玮师兄出国了，只能靠我自己做了，这时才感觉到真是力不从心呀。因为反应的中间产物是一种类似催泪瓦斯的东西，需要特别小心，我用过的烧瓶需要在通风柜里用碱水浸泡好长时间才能拿出来清洗。我记得一个用过的烧瓶已经浸泡了近两周了，我就从通风柜里拿出来开始清洗，哪里知道，我刚靠近烧瓶，就被里面残存的一点中间产物弄得涕泪横流，那真是眼泪哗哗的。连旁边的同学都被熏得不行，大家纷纷躲避，那时我才真正领略到这玩意的厉害。师兄告诉过我，如果这一烧瓶的产物洒了出来，整个逸夫技术科学楼都呆不住人，那罪过可就大了。从此，每次实验都胆战心惊的，生怕出现这种可怕的场面。至此，我萌生了放弃使用这种材料的念头。

但是在没有找到新的材料之前，我还一直继续使用这种材料，然而后续的文章评审意见成了"压倒我的最后一根稻草"，满满的 3 页，60 多条意见，把我的工作批得一无是处，并且说这个物质已经申请了专利，即使做研究也要经过他的允许。至此，我才下定决心，必须换一种新材料了。然而，由于当时对于脑组织修复的研究寥寥无几，选一种适用于脑组织修复的新材料谈何容易！我一下子陷入了苦恼之中，漫无目的地看着文献。有一天，我到孔祥东的宿舍里闲逛，看到他书桌上放着一本凌沛学教授编著的关于透明质酸的书，我顺手拿起来翻看，里面讲到了透明质酸凝胶的合成和应用，一个念头在我脑海里形成，能不能使用透明质酸水凝胶用于脑组织的修复呢？由于没有先例，心里也没有把握，因此我开始了围绕透明质酸用于脑组织损伤修复可行性的论证工作。我发现前人的研究说脑组织的细胞外基质主要是透明质酸，胶原的含量很低，我想使用与脑组织细胞外基质相似的物质应该能够促进脑组织损伤的修复，我对此有了信心。在一次与外科医生出身的余兴博士后的交谈中，谈到了我的想法，他说脑脊液里面也有很多透明质酸，应该是修复脑组织的理想材料。向崔老师汇报了我的想法,崔老师对我的想法很支持,并找到了时任首都医科大学校长的徐群渊教授合作开展研究,有了徐校长的支持和帮助,我的研究进入了"快车道"。我使用透明质酸水凝胶对大鼠脑损伤修复的研究得到了较好的结果,首次证明了透明质酸水凝胶具有良好的脑组织相容性。1 年以后,我的第一篇关于脑组织损伤修复的文章在 *Tissue Engineering* 上发表,迄今已被引用 100 余次。

当时关于中枢神经再生的机制研究有了突破性进展,发现了中枢神经再生的抑制因子 Nogo,在 *Nature* 上连续发了几篇文章,证实 Nogo 在抑制中枢神经再生中起着关键作用。因此,我就联想到能否将 Nogo 的抑制因子或者封闭抗体接枝到水凝胶中,利用缓释技术构建促进中枢神经再生的新系统。但是,实现这一想法面临的一个巨大的困难就是,当时无法获得封闭抗体,而且研究性的抗体量少且十分昂贵,不适合用于水凝胶的接枝。这个想法一直在心头,也思索着如何解决这一难题。在一次崔老师与徐群渊教授联合召开的讨论会上,我提出了这一想法,徐老师说这不是难事,首都医科大学宣武医院有一位制备抗体的高手,能够很容易实现 Nogo 抗体的快速制备。真是山重水复疑无路,柳暗花明又一村。几个月后,抗体便制备成功,而且效价很高。利用这个封闭性抗体,我们很快开始了透明质酸凝胶智能缓释系统的研制。首先与首都医科大学侯少平博士合作,验证了该缓释系统的体外诱导神经纤维定向再生的有效性。随后开始了体内试验,利用大鼠脑卒中模型,该缓释系统成功促进了神经再生和功能恢复。相关研究分别发表在 *Journal of Neuroscience Methods* 和 *Journal of Controlled Release* 上,这两篇文章的引用次数均达到 100 次左右。

总结我个人的经历,有以下想法:第一,博士选题不要有畏难情绪,要有敢闯的精神,因为博士生就是要围绕全新的课题进行开拓;第二,对于实验过程中遇到困难的实验方案,不要轻易放弃,可能以后就会想出克服困难的办法;第三,就是要与周围的人多交流,讨论你的想法,甚至是和不同学科的学者进行交流。生物材料本身就是一个跨学科的研究方向,需要多方面的知识和技能,多与相关学科人沟通一定会受益匪浅。

对于脑组织再生的未来研究方向,我没有过多的发言权。只是根据自己的经验提一点想法。脑是人体组织结构和功能最复杂的器官,迄今为止,科学家仍旧没有完全搞清其工作的机制。发达国家于 20 世纪 90 年代纷纷制定了脑科学研究的长远计划。美国 101 届国会通过一个议案,"命名 1990 年 1 月 1 日开始的 10 年为脑的 10 年"。1995 年夏,国际脑研究组织(International Brain Research Organization,IBRO)在日本京都举办的第 4 届世界神经科学大会上提议,把下一世纪(21 世纪)称为"脑的世纪"。欧共体成立了"欧洲脑的 10 年委员会"及脑研究联盟。日本推出了"脑科学时代"计划纲要,每年用于脑科学研发的预算总计约为 300 亿日元(约合 2.6 亿美元)。然而,10 年后,我们对脑的复杂高级认知功能的了解仍旧处在初始阶段，智慧的火花是如何产生的？让人束手无策的精神疾病是否有新的治疗路径？面对诸多挑战，2013年4月2日，奥巴马政府公布了新的脑计划，该计划旨在探索人类大脑工作机制、绘制脑活动全图，并最终开发出针对大脑疾病的疗法。随后，欧盟也提出了脑工程研究计划，我国最近也公布了脑研究计划。随着脑研究如火如荼地开展，组织工程和生物材料的研究能在其中发挥怎样的作用呢？最近有幸聆听了脑科学研究泰斗蒲慕明先生的讲座并与之交流，得到了许多有益的启发。鉴于大脑结构的极其复杂性，可以利用体外构建三维的脑组织，构建简化的脑模型进行研究。而最近的研究表明，利用诱导性多功能干细胞通过三维培养，可以得到类似大脑结构的三维组织。并且能够重复出小脑萎缩的疾病模型，而该模型尚无相应的动物模型。由此可见，利用水凝胶材料、干细胞以及三维生物打印技术有望构建出与体内更为近似的脑组织和结构，为揭示脑的工作机制提供良好的体外模型。

# 培养期间代表性文章

1. Tian W M, Hou S P, Ma J, Zhang C L, Xu Q Y, Lee I S, Li H D, Spector M, Cui F Z. Hyaluronic acid-poly-D-lysine-based three-dimensional hydrogel for traumatic brain injury. *Tissue Engineering*, 2005, 11 (3-4): 513-525.

**Abstract**　Brain tissue engineering in the postinjury brain represents a promising option for cellular replacement and rescue, providing a cell scaffold for either transplanted or resident cells. In this article, a hyaluronic acid (HA) -poly-D-lysine (PDL) copolymer hydrogel with an open porous structure and viscoelastic properties similar to neural tissue has been developed for brain tissue engineering. The chemicophysical properties of the hydrogel with HA : PDL ratios of 10 : 1, 5 : 1, and 4 : 1 were investigated by scanning electron microscopy (SEM) and X-ray photoelectron spectrometry. Neural cells cultured in the hydrogel were studied by phasecontrast microscope and SEM. The incorporation of PDL peptides into the HA-PDL hydrogel allowed for the modulation of neuronal cell adhesion and neural network formation. Macrophages and multinucleated foreign body giant cells found at the site of implantation of the hydrogel in the rat brain within the first weeks postimplantation decreased in numbers after 6 weeks, consistent with the host response to inert implants in numerous tissues. Of importance was the infiltration of the hydrogel by glial fibrillary acidic protein-positive cells-reactive astrocytes-by immunohistochemistry and the contiguity between the hydrogel and the surrounding tissue demonstrated by SEM. These findings indicated the compatibility of this hydrogel with brain tissue. Collectively, the results demonstrate the promise of an HA-PDL hydrogel as a scaffold material for the repair of defects in the brain.

引用次数: **100**

2. Tian W M, Zhang C L, Hou S P, Yu X, Cui F Z, Xu Q Y, Sheng S L, Cui H, Li H D. Hyaluronic acid hydrogel as Nogo-66 receptor antibody delivery system for the repairing of injured rat brain: in vitro. *Journal of Controlled Release*, 2005, 102 (1): 13-22.

**Abstract** Nogo-66 and NgR are important receptors inhibiting neuronal regeneration and therefore are targets for treating CNS injury. Antagonists of this receptor including blocking antibodies are potential therapeutic agents for CNS axonal injuries such as spinal cord and brain trauma. A new antibody (IgG) releasing system has been developed by covalently attaching IgG to the biodegradable hyaluronic acid (HA) hydrogel via the hydrolytically unstable hydrazone linkage, aiming to deliver the antibody of CNS regeneration inhibitors to the injured brain. In this paper we describe the synthesis, physico-chemical characteristics and test results of biological activity of antibody released from hyluronic acid hydrogel. To form the conjugates the antibody is attached to the polymer backbone using a condensation reaction between aldehyde group of the antibody and hydrazide group of the HA hydrogel. Furthermore, pH sensitive linkage-hydrozone has been formed between hydrogel and antibody. The amount of conjugated antibodies can reach 135 μg antibody/mg hydrogel in the dry state. At low pH, the antibodies released quite fast. However, the antibodies released much slower in neutral and alkaline environment. The bioactivity of antibody released from hydrogel was retained as demonstrated by indirect immunofluorescence technique.

引用次数: **68**

# 3.9　生物材料研究让我沉醉

## 孔祥东

浙江理工大学生命科学学院，杭州

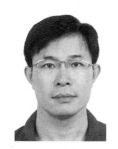

孔祥东，崔福斋教授 2001 级博士生，求学期间主要从事生物矿化、骨组织工程材料研究，博士论文题目为《丝素调制的磷酸钙生物矿化研究》。博士毕业以后于 2005 年 7 月到浙江理工大学生命科学学院工作，现为生命科学学院党委委员、副院长、教授。工作期间曾担任浙江理工大学党委办公室副主任兼校长办公室副主任，在国家科技部挂职锻炼两年，赴韩国延世大学做短期访问学者等。曾获浙江省优秀青年教师资助计划、浙江省 151 人才、浙江理工大学 521 拔尖人才项目支持，创办了浙江理工大学生物材料与海洋生物资源研究所（院级）、ZSTU-Dentium功能性生物材料与再生医学联合研究中心（校级）、杭州经济技术开发区"现代生物学"科普基地等。主要开展生物矿化与硬组织修复材料、肿瘤基因治疗的纳米药物载体、医用纺织品、蚕丝与贝壳等天然生物材料综合利用技术研究。已主持国家自然科学基金项目 3 项、浙江省自然科学基金项目等 15项，发表学术文章 70 余篇，申请中国发明专利 23 项。作为主要完成人获国家自然科学奖二等奖、浙江省科学技术奖一等奖、中冶集团科技进步奖二等奖、纺织工业联合会科学技术进步奖二等奖各 1 项。

到清华大学攻读博士学位并选择自己喜欢的研究方向实现了我梦寐以求的梦想。我先后从山东农业大学林学院、浙江大学动物科学学院、清华大学材料科学与工程系分别获得了学士、硕士和博士学位。人生求学经历的 3 个专业、3 所学校都给了我许多美好的回忆。其中在清华大学崔老师研究组的学习是我学术研究领域最为重要的学习阶段，所开展的生物材料交叉学科的研究让我产生了浓厚的兴趣。

由于博士之前的材料科学基础差，仅在读硕士期间从事过蚕丝蛋白材料研究，做过扫描电子显微镜分析、傅里叶变换红外光谱分析、差示扫描量热法材料表征分析，但是对于 X 射线衍射、透射电子显微术、选区电子衍射等深入的材料表征分析缺乏基础。在读博士期间，我知道崔老师已毕业的学生们都很优秀，许多同学在获得硕士、博士学位以后继续出国深造。材料科学与工程系对博士毕业要求发表 4 篇文章（两篇 SCI 收录，两篇核心期刊）。2001 年刚入学不久，崔老师在组会时开玩笑说："我们实验室以往博士大多发表 4 篇 SCI 文章，我不要求你们一定比他们强，但是你们一定不能比他们差吧？"能否从清华大学顺利毕业，对于我来讲是个非常大的挑战。

由于自己的材料科学基础差，我希望做一些偏向生物学的课题。我调研过转基因表达蚕丝蛋白的文章，做过蛞蝓黏液用于生物材料的可行性分析。最后的开题报告题目是《丝素蛋白微胶束固定化胰岛细胞用于 II 型糖尿病治疗的研究》。2003 年非典型性肺炎发生后的 4 月开始，因为与北京大学人民医院的合作变得非常不便，我最后的毕业论文题目变成了《丝素调制磷酸钙矿化的研究》，中间也经历了一些波折。

当时，研究组许多同学从事生物矿化模拟及硬组织相关生物材料研究，尤其是在胶原调制生物矿化方向，已在国际上发表了多篇有影响力的学术文章。当时，实验室选用的胶原主要是来自美国公司生产的牛胶原，可能存在一定的人畜共患疾病交叉感染的风险（尤其当时疯牛病的爆发为该类产品的医学应用蒙上了阴影）；另外，该类产品的价格也非常高。天然丝素蛋白的分子量为 30 万道尔顿左右，也是一种蛋白质，其生物相容性也非常优异，国际上已经有多篇关于蚕丝用于生物材料研究的报道。蚕丝蛋白的价格也相对便宜——1 g约 0.1~0.2 元左右。同时，蚕丝蛋白也是中国闻名世界并造福过全球的具有历史文化底蕴的传统纺织材料，其来源相对丰富。蚕丝若能应用于生物矿化材料，也是提升传统产业的一个重要应用方向，而且丝绸产业的废丝经过简单处理即可满足调制生物矿化的材料使用条件。在用丝素蛋白调制磷酸钙生物矿化研究的预备实验过程中，我发现水溶性丝素蛋白可显著影响磷酸钙生物矿化过程，含蛋白与不含蛋白的样品所制备的磷酸钙晶体的形貌迥异。于是，我又仔细研究了不同时间下丝素对低浓度磷酸钙（pH = 7.4）生物矿化的影响作用，并每隔 0.5 h 取样以备分析。

期间，我曾经在北京大学第三医院、清华大学的逸夫技术科学楼多次彻夜做过实验。当时，实验室内有一个人体骨骼模型，在瑟瑟寒风中，这具骨骼陪伴我度过一个又一个日夜。最后的分析结果表明实验很成功，含有丝素蛋白的磷酸钙溶液生长磷酸钙晶体的速度显著高于不含蛋白的对照组。在最后的选题以及开展实验研究的过程中，导师崔福斋教授给予了我精心的指导和耐心的帮助。

在那段时间，多次向身边的同学请教材料的表征及分析，最后又经过一遍又一遍的文章写作与修改，我学会了用 Endnote 处理数据，学会了用 Origin 作图，学会了用 Photoshop 处理图片。我感谢我的同窗：廖素三、王秀梅、马军、张伟、邹伟艳、彭奎庆等同学给予我的许多帮助，使我慢慢地融入了材料科学领域，并且掌握了从事材料科学研究所必备的分析工具与分析方法。

我在清华大学发表的第一篇文章 *Silk fibroin regulated mineralization of hydroxyapatite nanocrystals* 投稿时，王秀梅同学帮我做了最后的修改，崔老师建议我投到 *Journal of Crystal Growth* 上。文章投稿 1 个月后即被接收，评审人未要求做一个字的修改。评审人评价此文章为 "Important paper for biomineralization and importance of silk for crystallization of HA crystals"。截止到 2015 年底，该文章总被引用 110 多次，其中 SCI 文章引用 84 次，引用该文章的期刊包括 *Science*、*Nature Materials*、*Advanced Materials*、*Materials Science and Engineering：R：Reports*、*Biomaterials* 等。

这篇文章的发表给了我极大的信心和勇气，使我坚定了从事生物材料研究的决心，也为我今后从事交叉科学研究打下了坚实的基础。截至目前，我们尚难以在体外制备出与人类骨骼、牙齿在宏观与微观尺度全结构相同的合成材料，预示着该领域还有较大的研究空间。

## 培养期间代表性文章

Kong X D, Cui F Z, Wang X M, Zhang M, Zhang W. Silk fibroin regulated mineralization of hydroxyapatite nanocrystals. *Journal of Crystal Growth*, 2004, 270 (1-2)：197-202.

**Abstract**　In the present study, silk fibroin was employed to regulate the mineralization of hydroxyapatite（HA）nanocrystals. The calcium phosphate crystals precipitated in the aqueous solution of silk fibroin at pH 8 and room temperature. The depositions collected at different reaction time were detected by X-ray diffraction analysis to investigate the mineralization process of calcium phosphate. The results indicated that fibroin protein could significantly promote the crystal growth of HA. The formed HA crystals were also studied by Fourier transform infrared spectroscopy（FTIR）and transmission electron microscopy（TEM）. The FTIR results revealed that the HA crystals are carbonate-substituted HA and compounded with fibroin. There are strong chemical interactions between HA and fibroin protein, which can be derived from the blue shift of amide II peak（from the position of 1517−1539 $cm^{-1}$）. TEM images showed that the mineralized nanofibrils in the composites are rod like in shape with the diameter of about 2−3 nm. Selected area electron diffraction patterns from the composites exhibit polycrystalline rings, which were well indexed as the HA phase with 002 preferential orientations.

引用次数：**84**

# 3.10 长路漫漫的科学探索

马 军

华中科技大学生命科学与技术学院生物医学工程系，武汉

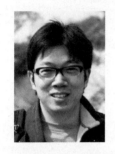

马军，1998年9月—2002年6月，清华大学材料科学与工程系，工学学士；2002年9月—2007年1月，清华大学材料科学与工程系，工学博士；2007年3月—2008年4月，新加坡 Nanomaterials Technology Pte. Ltd，研究助理；2008年10月—2010年9月，日本物质材料研究所，博士后研究员；2010年12月至今，华中科技大学生命科学与技术学院生物医学工程系，副教授。研究方向：① 针对骨、软骨和皮肤等组织特性，设计和制造新型多孔组织工程支架，用于组织再生和修复；② 多功能生物活性涂层材料，加速植入物与周围组织整合；③ 智能药物响应控释系统，增强植入材料或纳米材料在组织内的再生修复作用。

博士在读期间，从事神经元与材料的界面反应的研究，以化学腐蚀处理得到的纳米粗糙硅基片、仿生制备的静电自组装多层膜和微接触印刷图案等作为模型表面，研究了神经元细胞在体外培养条件下与材料的界面反应，以此来揭示材料表面特征与神经细胞相互作用的规律，研究开发在体外构建神经元网络的技术。

我进入崔老师的研究组后，先是做了一些模拟计算的研究工作，通过编写计算机程序，模拟碳纳米管在辐射粒子作用下的受损行为，这些研究工作和生物材料的关系并不大。经过一段时间的积累，我基本掌握了分子动力学模拟技术。有了这些基础，崔老师建议我尝试将分子动力学的研究手段用来研究生物矿化过程，这时候还有其他同学也参加进来。由于我个人投入的精力比较有限，当时在这个方面并未取得较大进展。在我到华中科技大学工作后，继续开展使用分子动力学方法研究胶原调制磷酸钙成核的研究，算是当年崔老师指导课题的延续。

在我确定攻读博士学位的时候，并没有明确选题。之所以没有将模拟计算

研究生物矿化作为博士研究课题，是有多方面原因的。一开始，我认真思考了选题的事情，觉得找准一个方向，选择一个有意义且可行的博士研究课题，应该慎重。崔老师建议我多看文献，多听报告，多看师兄、师姐的工作，这样才能做好选题工作。正好范师兄毕业离校，崔老师决定在新招收的研究生里找人继续发展范师兄建立起来的一些研究方向，尤其是在神经生物材料方面的研究。崔老师觉得我是一个不错的人选，他或许是觉得模拟计算的研究进展不够大，也不太适合作为一个博士研究课题，而神经生物材料在我们研究组刚刚起步，非常需要人手，因此，我算是被崔老师指定了一个课题。

选择神经科学与材料科学交叉的方向，我自己的兴趣也很大。自古以来，世人都很好奇，思考是怎么回事，而记忆又是怎么回事，神经系统如何从外界获取信息，又如何处理信息和存储信息。在这个领域有太多的未知，可以给科学研究提供大量的素材。自提出人机界面和脑机界面的研究计划以来，很多科学家都在这个领域雄心勃勃，希望有一天可以实现记忆的存储和读取。即便是简单的脑机界面，少许的信息互通，也能够给植物人、瘫痪或中风患者带来重生的可能。从这个意义上来讲，研究神经生物材料非常有意义，不仅适合作为重要的基础研究方向，而且还有巨大的潜在临床应用价值。将神经科学和生物材料进行交叉，作为我的博士课题主攻方向，应该非常容易找到有价值的研究内容。

那段时期，我们与首都医科大学徐群渊教授研究组的合作得到了进一步巩固。我、田维明与徐教授的博士生侯少平、刘丙方组成了合作小组。我们4个人常常一起研讨课题，开展研究工作。因为许多细胞实验和动物实验都在首都医科大学进行，如今的记忆中，我还深刻地记得我和田维明两人一大早赶公交，穿过大半个北京城去首都医科大学做一整天实验。那时候，对于动物解剖、原代神经细胞培养和动物损伤模型的研究，我们研究组还缺少经验。通过与徐教授团队的合作，我们快速在神经修复材料和神经界面材料的研究领域里跻身于一流水平，很快就有了一些积极的研究进展。在与徐教授团队的合作事宜上，崔老师态度一直非常坚决。他认为必须通过与一流团队的合作才能取得一流的研究成果。崔老师多次与我谈到，要想在神经生物材料领域做出成果，就必须加强与徐教授的合作。为了合作的事情，他还亲自前往首都医科大学，为我们解决实际问题，积极推动合作研究。在我攻读博士学位期间（2002—2007年），徐教授的团队对我们的合作课题给予了非常大的支持。

我当时搭档合作的伙伴是刘丙方，他是徐教授的在职博士生，拥有多年的神经细胞培养和免疫组化染色等经验，这些正好是我所欠缺的。在与首都医科大学合作的同时，我自己也尝试过在清华大学的实验室里面做一些神经细胞的培养实验，甚至还把侯少平和刘丙方请过来指导我的操作，结果是事倍功半。毕竟这些精细的实验操作技能需要多年的积累，非一日之功可以掌握熟练。经过了一年多的努力，我取得了一点进展，总结了一套监测神经细胞电位及其电势分布的显微研究方法，较为独立地写出了一篇文章并在 SCI 收录期刊上发表。那时候正好是博士一年级，这点成绩算不得什么，但是也给了我不少继续前进的动力，觉得做一些与生物科学交叉的研究并不是那么难。

经过崔老师点拨，我认识到了自身的诸多不足。如果要开展神经细胞与材料相互作用的研究，应该加强合作。通过合作，可以弥补自身的不足，加快自身的进步。在此之后，我与刘丙方的合作，进入到了更加密切的阶段。在合作中，我专注于设计和制造具有特殊结构的材料表面，而刘丙方则在细胞培养和免疫染色标记等方面做了不少工作。攻读博士学位的 4 年多时间里，我和刘丙方两人都从合作里面取得了超出我们预期的成绩，现在看起来，我们的合作是非常成功的，是典型的双赢。崔老师在合作研究这件事上，让我受益匪浅，让我切身体会到交叉学科的跨学科合作是非常重要的。

起初，捧着实验室积累下来的研究素材，我翻来覆去的琢磨如何重现前人的实验结果。我沿着硅表面纳米粗糙度的构造影响细胞黏附的研究方向探索了大概两年的时间，在这方面，我和刘丙方也取得了一些细胞与材料界面结构上的结果，发现神经细胞通过蛋白颗粒层在硅表面增加了黏附力。当时，我们实验室开发了一套共聚焦显微镜和原子力显微镜联用的技术，运用这项技术，我也做了一点关于神经细胞与硅界面的观测表征工作。虽然有了一些进步，但我们还是感觉在硅材料上的研究工作遇到了瓶颈。我们开始思考一些新的研究方向。查阅了许多国外同行的研究进展，我们想到是否可以通过电极阵列芯片来读取神经静息电位和动作电位，或者通过膜片钳等技术来研究神经电信号传递。正在迷茫的时候，崔老师提醒我们，这项研究的初衷是通过材料表面的图案设计，尤其是拓扑学的形貌设计来控制神经细胞的黏附，这个实验的直接目的就是为了调控神经细胞的黏附，获得体外有序神经网络，可以用来研究神经细胞之间的通讯方式。我们意识到，通过纳米尺度的形貌控制细胞黏附毕竟能力有限，这些因素很容易被外界的其他因素干扰，尤其是蛋白，所以我们猜测，通过蛋白的图案是否更加容易控制神经细胞黏附，进而实现神经网络的有序构建？

想到这里，刘丙方与我一拍即合，我们通过文献调研，立即调整了研究方向，将神经元网络的体外构建技术作为主攻方向。在汇报工作的时候，徐教授和崔老师都对我们的工作给予了肯定。我们选择了微接触印刷技术，这是美国哈佛大学的 Whitesides 教授提出的一系列软刻蚀技术中的一种，可以非常便捷地制造蛋白的图案。没过多久，我就掌握了微接触印刷技术，可以印刷一些简单的蛋白图案。刘丙方很快也将这个技术用在一些功能性蛋白的印刷上，我们相继尝试了层粘连蛋白和层粘连蛋白混合突触蛋白聚糖，在取得了一些初步进展后，我们确信通过微接触印刷获得的蛋白图案有更强的调控作用，能够在体外形成神经元的可控黏附，这距离我们成功构建神经元网络又近了一步。在这之后，我们也做了大量文献调研，最后发现电荷作用对神经元很敏感，就想到使用聚乙烯亚胺这种聚合物。将这种带正电荷的高分子用做印刷墨水，我们制备的神经网络结构很快就取得了积极的进展，得到了一个非常振奋的结果，也就是使用高分子聚乙烯亚胺图案调控的发育成熟的神经元网格。这个实验的结果也为我的博士论文画上了一个较为圆满的句号。

另外值得一提的是关于中枢神经修复水凝胶材料的研究。由于基于透明质酸的脑缺损修复水凝胶取得了较大的进展，我参加了中风模型的动物实验研究。崔老师对这个研究方向非常重视，常常组织小组讨论，并邀请了美国麻省理工大学的 Myron Spector 教授到北京，参与指导我们的工作。通过一系列体外研究试验发现，我们设计的携带 Nogo-66 抗体的水凝胶材料可以诱导神经细胞生长，为进一步作为脑缺损修复提供了佐证。起初的这些实验，只是解决了组织修复的一些问题，并未涉及到功能修复。随后，我们设计了一个脑卒中的缺血损伤大鼠模型，也就是俗称的中风。为了这个实验，我们几人在这个动物实验里面都投入了长达数年的时间。由于行为学动物实验非常复杂，而且工作量巨大。最终，我们取得了一些积极的结果，但是并不如预期的理想。可能是对于行为学动物实验的经验不足，导致统计学数据的意义不是非常明显。这也给我们一个启示，那就是对待实验结果，必须做好各方面的准备。在 Myron Spector 教授的帮助下，我们几经周折，将这个结果发表在 *Biomedical Materials* 上。这篇关于水凝胶材料用做脑缺血模型损伤修复的实验研究报道，发表至今还不断被人引用，也算是我们在神经修复材料领域的一个阶段性重要成果。在此之后，我们做了一些调整，将研究方向转向了更加基础的一些领域，希望可以通过更基础的实验来揭示神经细胞与材料的作用机制，例如，当时我们注意到干细胞的研究进展，提出通过材料特性诱导干细胞分化的研究思路。通过更加简单的模型材料界面来研究揭示神经细胞和神经系统与材料的相互作用，这之后的研究工作就由魏岳腾和任永娟等人继续。

在我攻读博士期间，在神经生物材料的研究团队中，除个人的科研工作外，崔老师还让我组织新加入的研究生，协助指导他们的研究工作。在崔老师的安排下，我还担任实验室大型设备管理员多年。回想起当年在崔老师身边得到的那些锻炼，感觉受益匪浅。总结多年的科学研究工作，我有两点感想：其一，交叉领域的研究需要合作，取长补短，方能有所作为，这也是所谓的站在巨人的肩膀上的道理；其二，研究的创新需要思维的碰撞和探索，更需要积极的态度和脚踏实地地工作，只有踏踏实实地做实验，才能有所进步。对于崔老师这次提到的"温故而知创新"的主题，我也颇有感触。当时，清华大学图书馆有一个外文原版书架，有许多经典的材料科学和生命科学书籍，我几乎是一本本的读过去的。通过这些知识的积累，为科学研究打下了基础，很多解决问题的想法都来自这些平日的阅读中。

写下上面这些文字后，我翻开当年的笔记本，从渐渐淡去的笔迹中，我觉得当年的努力都是值得的。科学探索长路漫漫，吾将上下而求索。

## 培养期间代表性文章

Ma J, Liu B F, Xu Q Y, Cui F Z. AFM study of hippocampal cells cultured on silicon wafers with nano-scale surface topograph. *Colloids And Surfaces B: Biointerfaces*, 2005, 44 (2-3): 152-157.

**Abstract**    The rat hippocampal cells were selected as model to study the interaction between the neural cells and silicon substrates using atomic force microscopy (AFM). The hippocampal cells show tight adherence on silicon wafers with nano-scale surface topograph. The lateral friction force investigated by AFM shows significant increase on the boundary around the cellular body. It is considered to relate to the cytoskeleton and cellular secretions. After ultrasonic wash in ethanol and acetone step by step, the surface of silicon wafers was observed by AFM sequentially. We have found that the culture leftovers form tight porous networks and a monolayer on the wafers. It is concluded that the leftovers overspreading on the silicon substrates are the base of cell adherence on such smooth inert surfaces.

引用次数：**16**

# 3.11 学研到产业实现的几点心得

## 胡 堃

北京印刷学院，北京

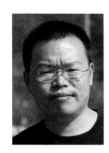

胡堃，高级工程师，全国外科植入物和矫形器械标准化技术委员会组织工程医疗器械产品分技术委员会委员。博士培养时间：2003 年 9 月—2007 年 7 月。

作为一名理工科从业者，仅从自己的从业过程中的感触，记录下对产学研一体化在创新创业中的重要性的认知。这也是崔老师交代的特殊任务：别的师兄弟谈学术研究，我谈产业转化经历，也算是扬长避短吧。学研是产业的动力源泉，而产学研一体化则是生产力不断进步的发动机，是社会进步过程中人这一环节的重要培养间。

### 1. 我的就业经历

学业结束的时候面临出国还是国内就业的选择，这时，我的导师崔福斋教授邀请我参加公司的管理，在犹豫之时，一直尊敬的董何彦教授告诉我说："学习、研发等活动的终极目的是产业，产业的最高要求是标准化，我们国家在这方面需要勇敢的从业者，现在选择从事产业化工作是很好的时机和机会，也会是将来良好的发展方向。"那是 10 多年前，现在想起来，确实如此。因为从事的项目是实验室的成果向产业化的转化，中间经历了标准的制定、工艺化的确定、人员团队建设、产品的型检和注册等一系列的过程，其实也是产学研结合的过程。有阶段性成功的喜悦，也有阶段性没有结果的沮丧。

### 2. 经历中的感触

首先，产学研是一个整体，不可分割。产学研主要针对的是应用性学科，重要的就是要产业化，但产业化就有其固有的实现方法。以植入性医疗器械为例，研究的时候，要清楚材料的成分和结构，要有创新，以便发文章、申请专利等；但结果的获得带有很强的偶然性，实验可以重复，但没有标准化、流程化，而后者就是产品产业化要具备的基本要素。大学和研究院的教授作为创业者的主体，本身是学研的带头者，需要加强对产业过程规律规则的认知。

其次，产学研过程中，团队建设的完整性不可忽视。学研团队从事产业化，最容易忽略的地方就是哪里重要哪里有人，哪个事情重要就主要做哪个事情，道理上容易接受，但若是健康公司的发展就需要完备团队，岗位设置到位，即使没有那么多从业者，也要尽可能把必要的岗位设置好，身兼多职也要建设好管理体系。

再次，质量管理体系十分重要，要一开始就建设成可实操的体系。其定义如下：质量管理是在质量方面指挥和控制组织的协调活动，通常包括制定质量方针、目标以及质量策划、质量控制、质量保证和质量改进等活动。实现质量管理的方针目标，有效地开展各项质量管理活动，必须建立相应的管理体系，这个体系就叫做质量管理体系。它可以有效进行质量改进。对医疗器械生产者来讲，质量管理体系尤为重要，从国家监管层面来讲也是重点监控内容，产品的注册、生产、销售、市场等都有具体的法规要求和控制，对企业来讲，也是通过质量管理体系的有效运作，实现对产品质量的把控，实现市场流通中产品的安全有效性的保证。而现在体系的要求中，对于产品实现过程的学研部分的要求越来越多，分量越来越重要，包括产品制作机理、工艺实现的方法、实现有效性的机理、安全性的保证等，这些都需要学研来解决，利用科研的力量和经历去实现问题的解答，研究得越透彻，越容易实现产业化的清晰化和保证效率。例如一款止血材料的产品，需要研究这个止血材料的成分组成和结构；需要研究这个止血材料的止血机理、是否降解、降解周期和成分；产品的生物安全性指标，包括细胞毒、遗传毒等。这些都可以在研究阶段进行透彻的研究，并有公开发表文章，就会省却很多产业化过程的验证工作（当然工艺确定后的正常验证流程和检验流程都要进行），也便于产品的审批上市。

最后，就是产学研从业者的自由和利益保障，政策对于创业的支持等非常关键和重要。曾几何时，产学研结合的项目，科研院所和大学的教授不能直接从业，间接的过程往往就会使得项目走形。幸好的是，国务院近日印发《关于进一步做好新形势下就业创业工作的意见》（下称《意见》）中以保留体制内身份和待遇三年为优惠条件，鼓励他们离岗创业。对体制内人员走出去创业给予政策支持。《意见》指出，随着我国经济发展进入新常态，就业总量压力依然存在，结构性矛盾更加凸显。必须着力培育大众创业、万众创新的新引擎，实施更加积极的就业政策，把创业和就业结合起来，以创业创新带动就业。鼓励利用财政性资金设立的科研机构、普通高校、职业院校，通过合作实施、转让、许可和投资等方式，向高校毕业生创设的小微企业优先转移科技成果。完善科技人员创业股权激励政策，放宽股权奖励、股权出售的企业设立年限和盈利水平限制。在这样的环境中，体制内工作在一线的科研人员可身无顾及地加入到"大众创业、万众创新"的创业潮中，在体制内的工作不受影响的前提下，又可以把自主研发的创新型项目亲自推向产业化，与自我的利益挂钩，这必将提高创业成功率，成为中国经济转型升级的重要力量。

2014 年，科技部科技型中小企业技术创新基金管理中心又发布了《关于做好 2014 年度科技型中小企业技术创新基金项目组织推荐准备工作的通知》（国科企金〔2014〕2 号）。对科技型中小企业特别是小微企业的产品研发给予支持。支持方式包括无偿资助、贷款贴息。从而营造出适合高层次人才创业创新的政策环境。

3. 产学研过程中的感触

我们知道，创业是创业者对自己拥有的资源或通过努力能够拥有的资源进行优化整合，从而创造出更大经济或社会价值的过程。这个过程中优化整合自己的资源是可控的，但努力要拥有的资源就是对创业者最大的吸引，这里面有人力资源、成本优势、环境卫生、扶持政策、政策的持久保持等。

习近平总书记鼓励医疗器械行业："医疗设备是现代医疗业发展的必备手段，现在一些高端医疗设备基层买不起、老百姓用不起，要加快高端医疗设备国产化进程，降低成本，推动民族品牌企业不断发展，你们的事业大有可为。"相信医疗器械高值耗材研发生产经营企业，可在国家和地方政策的支持下，产学研一体化的推动下，有序加快进行项目产业化，并作为高增长型企业快速成长，从而催生经济社会发展新动力。

# 培养期间代表性文章

Hu K, Lv Q, Cui F Z, Feng Q L, Kong X D, Wang H L, Huang L Y, Li T. Biocompatible fibroin blended films with recombinant human-like collagen for hepatic tissue engineering. *Journal of Bioactive and Compatible Polymers*, 2006, 21（1）: 23-37.

**Abstract** Recombinant human-like collagen（RHLC）was blended with fibroin to prepare a novel biocompatible film as a scaffold material for hepatic tissue engineering applications. Solution blending was used to incorporate RHLC with silk fibroin to enhance the blend films biocompatibility and hydrophilicity while maintaining elasticity. FTIR and XRD analysis indicated that hydrogen bonds had formed between fibroin and RHLC, while SEM microscopy data confirmed that homogeneous microstructures were still retained after the introduction of RHLC with fibroin. Contact angle measurements indicated that the hydrophilicity of the fibroin/RHLC films was greater after RHLC was added. The elongation at break in the wet state was not markedly changed after blending the recombinant human-like collagen, which implied that flexibility was maintained. The proliferation and viability of the cell cultures on fibroin/RHLC films were significantly enhanced compared to pure fibroin films or tissue culture plates.

引用次数: 31

# 3.12 胶原矿化机理及骨修复材料研究

## 王 玉

斯伦贝谢油田技术服务公司，北京

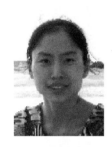

王玉，2003 级直博生，研究方向为矿化胶原形成机理及用于骨修复材料的研究。毕业后在斯伦贝谢油田技术服务公司先后从事测井工程师、软件测试工程师及软件技术支持工程师。

本人博士期间的研究课题包括矿化胶原形成机理及骨修复材料两方面。研究方向的确立是基于生物材料实验室崔福斋教授研究组以往的研究工作。

生物矿化（biomineralization），是指在一定条件下，在生物体的不同部位，以各种作用方式，在有机基质和细胞的参与下，无机元素从环境中选择性地在特定的有机基质上形核、生长和相变而转变为结构高度有序的生物矿物的过程。生物矿化区别于一般矿化的一个显著特征是，它通过有机大分子和无机矿物离子在界面处的相互作用，从分子水平控制无机矿物的析出，从而使生物矿物具有特殊的高级结构和组装方式。生物矿化现象在自然界中广泛存在，目前已知的生物矿物超过 60 种，其中含钙的矿物最多，占生物矿物总数的一半。长期以来，缺损骨骼的修复一直是骨研究领域的重要任务。以往，骨的修复主要依赖于金属替代材料和自体骨移植，骨的仿生制备直到近 20 年来才成为可能。如何按人体骨组织的结构与成分，制备具有与人骨类似的成分和显微结构的框架材料，使之与活体成骨细胞或骨生长因子复合，研制出具有良好的骨传导性能和骨诱导性能的骨修复材料，是一项具有十分重要科学意义和现实价值的研究课题。生物材料实验室多年来致力于骨骼矿化机理的研究并将其应用于胶原调制羟基磷灰石制备仿生骨修复材料。骨属于胶原-磷酸钙复合系统，是一个复杂的天然生物矿化系统。其主要组成是水、有机物和无机盐等。有机物中 90% 以上为 I 型胶原，还有少量的非胶原性蛋白、多糖、脂类等。无机盐中主要为磷酸钙类。本人在博士期间研究了天然胶原、重组胶原调制磷酸钙生长的生物矿化过程的机理，并在此基础上仿生制备了矿化重组胶原基骨修复材料，解决了以往动物源性胶原基骨材料的病毒隐患等安全问题。并进一步提高了材料的生物相容性，赋予材料骨诱导性，获得了具有广阔市场前景的新型骨修复材料。

生物矿化机理研究是制备具有优异性能的仿生材料的基础，研究生物矿化过程中胶原和磷酸钙的相互作用对于仿生骨材料的制备至关重要。我们的研究指出，在磷酸钙发生非晶/晶体转变及晶体成熟过程中，胶原发生明显的构象变化，以适应晶体的形成和长大。结合以往的研究，进一步对体外胶原矿化全过程进行了阐述，促进了对体内生物矿化的理解。基于这些理解，使用自组装的方法制备了纳米羟基磷灰石/胶原复合材料。按照这种方法得到的材料从成分上和结构上都和天然骨有着很大的相似性。相对于传统胶原/羟基磷灰石复合材料来说，由于此材料中羟基磷灰石是纳米相，材料具有更好的生物学性能，这使得它在骨替代材料方面得到广泛应用。但这些研究中所用的胶原主要提取自动物组织，应用于植入材料存在免疫反应、交叉感染病毒等安全问题（例如疯牛病），越来越受到人们的关注。重组人源性胶原技术的发展为我们提供了可靠的、可控的、化学成分明确的不含动物组织成分的纯化类人胶原。但重组胶原是否可以调制磷酸钙的形核生长，我们是否可以按生物自组装的思路制备仿生的重组胶原/羟基磷灰石复合材料仍需探讨。通过对重组胶原调制磷酸钙矿化的研究，我们证明重组胶原上的羟基可与钙离子配位，成为矿物形核位点，调制纳米级磷酸钙形核生长，得到仿生的矿化重组胶原，为制备仿生的矿化重组胶原基骨材料提供了理论根据。

基于以上的理论研究，我们首次用仿生的矿化重组胶原代替天然动物源性胶原制备出新型骨修复框架材料。该材料的成分和结构均与天然骨相似，通过体外细胞实验和体内动物实验，证明其具有良好的生物相容性和骨传导性，可以达到与动物源性胶原基骨材料相同的效果。而重组胶原避免了动物源性胶原的安全隐患，使新材料具有更高的安全性能，有望替代天然胶原基骨材料而成为骨修复的优选材料。

我们制备的重组胶原基骨修复材料成分包括重组胶原、纳米羟基磷灰石和聚乳酸，前两者与天然骨十分相似，具有良好的生物相容性，用于成型的聚乳酸与其他人工合成高分子材料相比也具有较好的生物相容性和优异的力学强度，并且已经通过美国 FDA 批准，可以植入人体。但是，作为组织工程框架材料，在一些方面仍不够理想。第一，由于聚乳酸为疏水材料，该框架材料的疏水性较强，不利于细胞在材料表面黏附和铺展；第二，聚乳酸的生物相容性无法和胶原、透明质酸等天然生物材料相比，而这直接关系到正常细胞的增殖和组织的形成。卵磷脂是具有亲油性和亲水性的双亲分子，同时又是人体细胞膜的重要组成部分，是一种有利于细胞和组织生长的天然生物材料，极适宜在体内降解，无毒性，无免疫原性。卵磷脂是脂溶性物质，可溶于脂溶性溶剂，这使得卵磷脂可以和聚乳酸通过溶液共溶方式混合，从而引入框架材料内部，从材料整体性能上提高生物相容性。经过我们的实验研究，在材料制备过程加入适量的双亲性卵磷脂可以显著提高材料的亲水性，更有利于细胞在材料上的黏附和增殖。混合材料在生物体内不引起显著的免疫排斥反应，具有更高的生物相容性。

生长因子有助于诱导宿主实质细胞的长入，并能促进移植细胞更好地形成再生组织。通过复合生长因子有效提高材料的生物活性也是骨修复研究的热点。骨形成蛋白BMP作为最有效的成骨诱导活性物质，已被广泛应用在骨缺损修复及骨折愈合的研究中。其中BMP-2的诱导成骨能力最强。但天然的BMP-2不仅数量有限，而且混入载体中有许多副作用。运用转基因技术制备的基因重组BMP-2也存在转染效率低、表达时间较短及病毒载体的潜在致癌性等缺点。华中科技大学同济医学院附属协和医院骨科郑启新教授、郭晓冬教授根据BMP-2的抗原决定族用固相多肽合成法合成含24个氨基酸的寡肽—BMP-2活性多肽。它可以发挥与BMP-2类似的独特的骨诱导活性，较易用多肽合成仪大规模制备，有效克服了国内外用基因工程技术制备时工艺复杂、价格昂贵及安全性隐患等缺点。我们的研究表明复合了BMP-2活性多肽的骨材料，在大鼠异位成骨实验中可引起肌肉组织内的异位成骨，并存在量效关系。对于大鼠5 mm全层颅骨缺损可以有效促进骨再生，在20周时达到愈合，材料基本完全降解。重组胶原基骨材料与动物源性胶原基骨材料相比效果无显著差异。

本人在对天然胶原、重组胶原调制磷酸钙生长的生物矿化过程机理研究的基础上，仿生制备了矿化重组胶原基骨修复材料，解决了以往动物源性胶原基骨材料的病毒隐患等安全问题。并通过复合卵磷脂和生长因子，进一步提高了材料的生物相容性，赋予材料骨诱导性，获得了具有广阔市场前景的新型骨修复材料。重组胶原由于具有动物源胶原蛋白无法比拟的优势，可以更广泛地应用于医学领域。随着基因重组技术的不断成熟，重组胶原有望成为替代天然胶原的安全可靠材料，大量应用于仿生骨材料的制备与研发。重组生长因子也将随着基因重组技术的发展和生长因子研究的深入而不断完善和改进，为仿生材料的改性提供更多的选择和裨益。

祝愿我国生物材料事业蒸蒸日上，人才辈出，跻身于国际领先地位。

## 培养期间代表性文章

Wang Y, Cui F Z, Zhai Y, Wang X M, Kong X D, Fan D D. Investigations of the initial stage of recombinant human-like collagen mineralization. *Materials Science and Engineering: C*, 2006, 26 (4): 635-638.

**Abstract** To found the theoretical foundation for applying recombinant human-like collagen (RHLC) to bone tissue engineering, the initial stage of RHLC mineralization was studied for the first time by using Fourier Transform Infrared Spectrometry (FTIR), Scanning Electron Microscopy (SEM) and Transmission Electron Microscopy (TEM). SEM images showed that samples of RHLC/calcium phosphate were spongy. TEM images and Selected Area Electron Diffraction (SAED) exhibited that the RHLC fibers in the mineralized samples were surrounded by HA nanocrystals. By comparing the FTIR spectra of RHLC, RHLC/$Ca^{2+}$ and RHLC/calcium phosphate, it was observed that the peak for amide I shifted to a lower wavenumber indicating that there is chemical interaction between carbonyl groups of RHLC and calcium ions. These results are consistent with previous studies of natural collagen mineralization. It is reasonable to conclude that RHLC can regulate the deposition of HA nanocrystals and may be used in bone tissue engineering.

引用次数：**46**

# 3.13  目标明确，开放合作

## 李　艳

东南大学生物科学与医学工程学院，南京

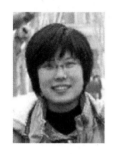

李艳，2003 年，于四川大学生物医学工程专业取得学士学位，同年师从崔福斋教授直接攻读博士学位，博士论文《bFGF 和 BMSCs 在骨再生修复中的应用研究》获得 2008 年清华大学优秀博士毕业论文二等奖。2008 年 7 月，博士毕业后进入东南大学生物科学与医学工程学院从事教学及科研工作至今，主要从事医用纳米材料的生物学效应研究。

晃眼间，博士毕业已经七八年了，读博时的种种，选择课题时的迷茫，实验受挫时的灰心，文章发表时的喜悦，至今还历历在目。在恩师崔福斋教授 70 大寿之际，应师兄、师姐的号召，还工作在科研前线上的我撰此文，在为恩师贺寿的同时，也为自己的博士生涯做总结留念，为自己以后的科研探索之旅拨开迷雾，呈现路径。

我是 2003 年从四川大学生物医学工程专业本科毕业，有幸推研成为崔老师的直博生，跟随崔老师开始科学研究之路。最开始的尝试是我的本科毕业设计课题，题目是《纳米晶胶原基骨材料/骨系细胞的相互作用》。第一次接触骨修复材料、组织工程这样的概念，第一次了解科研人员为躯体创伤病人的康复所做出的种种努力，也慢慢筑建了一直到现在我所理解的应用基础科学研究的意义，种种尝试，只为造福人类，造福社会。

博士研究生期间，崔老师引领我在更好地促进骨的再生修复方面做出了很多尝试和努力。尽管读博初期，受当时一些热门文章的吸引，我也走过一些弯路。崔老师跟我深切地谈过一次话，第一，问我所做工作的意义是什么，做出的材料的用途是什么。第二，跟我讲了我们研究组一直以来努力的方向，从牙齿骨骼的分级结构研究开始，到尝试揭开生物矿化的机理，再到相关硬组织修复材料的实验室仿生制备，众多师兄、师姐在此道路上尝试的工作及取得的成果。第三，跟我讲了科学研究的意义。我们所做工作，目的不是为了发表一篇影响因子多么高的文章，之后再无下文，而是要做对促进人类健康生活"有用"的材料和后续产品，这才是生物材料的终极意义。直到今天，我一直很庆幸自己在崔老师的引领下进入生物材料研究这个领域，在改善提高人类生命质量这个明确目标的指引下，在前人所做的种种贡献基础上，尽自己所能，取得哪怕是技术上的一个小小进步，也是我所承担工作的价值所在。

之后的日子，顺理成章，以实验室已经开发出的矿化胶原基骨修复材料（nHAC/PLA）作为实验对象，研究其作为框架材料与骨髓间充质干细胞（bone marrow stem cells, BMSCs）、成骨诱导剂地塞米松和抗坏血酸以及碱性成纤维细胞生长因子（basic fibroblast growth factor, bFGF）的体外复合，以复合材料的体内外成骨效应作为评价手段，改善材料的骨修复能力，力求为相关骨缺损的临床治疗提供新型解决办法和实验依据，这些一步步丰富了我的博士论文内容。在此，我想着重讲述的是基体材料与 bFGF 的复合。

框架材料、种子细胞和生长因子是组织工程的三要素。当时，我已经将地塞米松和抗坏血酸成功地引入 nHAC/PLA 材料内部，体外释放后可以诱导 BMSCs 向成骨细胞分化。而在骨的再生修复过程中，除了成骨定向分化，细胞的增殖以及后续的功能实现也很重要，bFGF 正好可以担任这样的角色。它能够促进相关细胞的增殖与分化，加快骨组织的生成。有很多研究者将其与各类载体材料复合，用于体内骨或软骨组织的修复。要想达到良好的使用效果，bFGF 最好能从载体中持续缓慢释放，这就涉及蛋白与载体复合的问题。蛋白的复合方法主要包括物理吸附、静电自组装以及化学交联等。而将载体材料浸入到含蛋白的超饱和钙磷盐溶液中，利用蛋白与磷酸钙的共沉淀，将蛋白固定在载体表面新形成的磷灰石层中，因为这种方法简便易行，也吸引了不少研究者的关注。

作为崔老师的学生，我赴韩国首尔参与崔老师跟延世大学的 In-Seop Lee 教授的合作交流，为期半年。崔老师和 Lee 教授共同的朋友，日本产业技术综合研究所（Advanced Industrial Science and Technology, AIST）的 Atsuo Ito 博士在医用磷酸钙表面复合不同种类的蛋白方面做了很多工作，其中非常吸引人的是他们采用 3 种医用临床注射液，根据不同比例混合制备饱和磷酸钙溶液，再将蛋白溶解于混合溶液中，将蛋白共沉淀于材料表面新形成的钙磷盐层中。他们所采用的 3 种溶液是日本医院的医用处方注射液，可以保证其用于人体的安全性。我们当时想借鉴一下他们的方法，于是跟 Ito 博士联系，第一次是通电话，Ito 博士热心友好，应该是顾虑到我的英语听力水平，语速缓慢，发音清晰，对我提出的问题毫无保留地予以回答，最后留了他的 e-mail 地址，让我跟他写信联系，没有丝毫不耐烦。甚至在以后的 e-mail 中，将他们之前的技术资料，例如，3 种溶液在不同配比情况下所得混合溶液中各离子的浓度，以及实验中要注意的小细节、小窍门，全都毫无保留地以文档形式发送给了我。之后开会时跟 Ito 博士见过几次面，才发现原来早在 2005 年武汉召开的一次国际会议上就听过他的报告。直到今天，我一直对 Ito 博士心存感激敬佩之情，温和儒雅、学者风范是对其最好的诠释。其实在跟他通完第一次电话之后，我就对课题的前景充满了信心。科研道路上，前辈的无私热心无疑会赋予我们不畏难的勇气和力量。在以后的日子里，我一直以 Ito 博士作为模范，对于科研问题保持开放探讨的态度，也希望将来的自己能给别人类似的帮助。

之后我顺利确定了溶液配比，成功将 bFGF 固定于 nHAC/PLA 材料表面，体外持续缓慢释放，并能够促进表面接种前成骨细胞的增殖生长。与此同时，我们还选定了钛基牙科种植体作为基体材料，在其表面复合 bFGF，提高其植入体内的骨整合性。由于其良好的耐腐蚀性、耐磨性等机械性能，钛及钛合金成为迄今临床应用广泛的植入材料，用于制作人工关节、骨内固定器材、人工牙根以及下颌骨和颅骨的缺损修复等。但它同时也存在着金属材料通有的局限性，例如生物活性差、缺乏骨诱导作用、与周围组织无强有力的化学结合、愈合时间较长等，难以满足临床愈合快、骨结合强度高等要求。为了改善其生物活性，提高其骨整合性，研究者们开展了大量工作对其表面进行改性研究。我们的思路是将阳极氧化处理与电子束沉积磷酸钙涂层相结合，构建出一种钛/磷酸钙复合植入物，随后通过溶液浸入，在复合体表面进一步复合 bFGF。

这个实验一直存在着种种困难。基体材料钛是我之前并不熟悉的，其各种表面处理方法对我来说也是陌生的，用前述溶液共沉淀 bFGF 也并不成功，当时我还身处异国，面对实验室的微弧氧化设备，心情难以言述。也是那个时候，对于科研有了更深入的理解，有几件事情对我影响至今。其一，数据就是数据，不分好坏。这是当时我在跟崔老师和 Lee 教授汇报工作时，总是很沮丧地讲实验结果不好而获得的良言。其二，科研就是探查未知真相，实事求是。当时去旁听过几次学术会议，有好几个研究者，也是力图提高牙科植入物的骨整合性，他们做了很多尝试，但最后展现的植入效果并未有提高，看到他们在台上或平静或仍然激情地阐述相关结论，我彻底领悟科研的真正内涵。其三，实验就是要不断尝试，山重水复疑无路，柳暗花明又一村。如前所述，用 Ito 的方法固定 bFGF 失败。由于饱和磷酸钙溶液中含有 $NaHCO_3$，随着孵育时间的推移，溶液中会持续释放 $CO_2$ 气体，从而造成溶液 pH 值的不断增大，极易形成磷酸钙沉淀。样品浸入混合溶液 2 h 后，表面就会形成一层肉眼可见的薄膜，且此薄膜在清洗条件下就极易脱落。这可能是由于溶液中自发形成的磷酸钙沉淀过多，开线过快，而钛/磷酸钙复合体不像之前所用 nHAC/PLA 材料，多孔结构使其本身就有很好的吸附效果，因此，难以与新生成磷酸钙层牢固结合所致。我总结整理了能够查阅到的文献中曾经出现的模拟体液，列表分析其无机离子浓度的异同，一一尝试，最后发现恰恰是我们常用的杜氏磷酸盐缓冲液（Dulbecco's phosphate buffered saline，DPBS），可以用来很好地在钛基材料表面覆盖的磷酸钙层上固定 bFGF。方法确定后，我们又顺利完成了后续的体内外成骨效应评价，部分结果也即后面所列文章，最终发表在 *Biomaterials* 上。在这里，我还想对 Lee 教授的博士生，现在首尔科技大学工作的 In-hoo Han 博士致以谢意，感谢他在试剂订购、仪器预约方面所给予的帮助，以及在日常生活中所给予的温情。

时光飞逝，一晃而过，而今博士毕业参加工作已经 7 年多。这期间工作进展颇为缓慢，研究方向也时有不定，但并不敢轻言放弃。那些曾经接受过的科研训练、恩师的教导、前辈的无私、同门的友爱，时时在心，鞭策着我。因为是自己的博士课题工作，对于骨的再生修复也一直保持着关注，私以为在以下几个方面尚有较大空间的发展：

（1）原理探索方面：骨再生的生理基础，包括成骨细胞、破骨细胞的生物功能、信号途径；骨矿物沉积过程中各种蛋白质多糖等分子的作用。

（2）材料的制备修饰：新型优异骨材料的开发以及后续的功能修饰。

（3）应用研究方面：针对特定应用，发展关键技术，例如组织工程复合体的构建技术、靶细胞的操纵技术等，达到真正促进临床骨再生修复的目的。

# 培养期间代表性文章

1. Cui F Z, Li Y, Ge J. Self-assembly of mineralized collagen composites. *Materials Science & Engineering R：Reports*，2007，57（1-6）：1-27.

**Abstract**    This paper presents a review of the current understanding of the structure，self-assembly mechanisms，and properties of mineralized collagen fibril composites in connective tissues，such as in lamellar bones，woven bones，zebrafish skeletal bone，and ivory. Recent work involving biomimetic synthesis of new materials with the structure of mineralized collagen is described. The focus in the paper is mainly on materials containing type I collagen，with mineralization by Ca-P crystals although some other systems are also described. Investigation and simulation of naturally occurring fibril structures can offer some new ideas in the design and fabrication of new functional materials，for applications such as bone grafts or for use as scaffolds in tissue engineering and biomimetic engineering materials. The development of bone grafts based on the mineralization of self-assembled collagen fibrils in vivo and in vitro is an active area of research. This kind of bone graft composite has already shown great promise and success in clinical applications，on account of its compositional and structural similarity to autologous bone. It is suggested that future work in this should focus on both basic theoretical aspects as well as the development of applications. In particular issues including control of morphology，incorporation of foreign ions, interaction with biomolecules, and the assembly of organic and inorganic phases are all still not well understood. In the area of applications, the design of composite materials with a hierarchical structure closer to that of natural hard tissues, and the synthesis of bone grafts and tooth regenerative materials, as well as biomimetic functional materials, are areas currently being examined by many research groups.

引用次数: **140**

2. Li Y, Lee I S, Cui F Z, Choi S H. The biocompatibility of nanostructured calcium phosphate coated on micro-arc oxidized titanium. *Biomaterials*, 2008, 29 (13): 2025-2032.

**Abstract**　To achieve improved osseointegration, there have been many efforts to modify the surface composition and topography of dental implants. Recently, the anodic oxidation treatment of titanium (Ti) has attracted a great deal of attention. Meanwhile, calcium phosphate is commonly applied to metallic implants as a coating material for fast fixation and firm implant-bone attachment on the account of its demonstrated bioactive and osteoconductive properties. In the present study, anodized surface and calcium phosphate deposition by electron beam evaporation were combined. Nanostructured calcium phosphate film was deposited on the micro-arc oxidized Ti. New apatite layer formed easily on the coated film when incubating in DPBS solution at 37 ℃. By adding basic fibroblast growth factor (bFGF) in the DPBS solution, the bFGF could be immobilized in the newly formed apatite layer. The coated film enhanced osseointegration of Ti implants in vivo.

引用次数: **89**

# 3.14　学科交叉促进科研创新

## ——祝贺崔福斋教授 70 寿辰

### 王程越

辽宁医学院附属第二医院，锦州

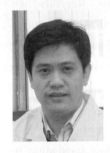

王程越，1999 年，于辽宁医学院口腔系取得学士学位，同年于锦州市中心医院口腔科工作；2004 年，于中国医科大学口腔医学院攻读博士学位，师从艾红军教授。期间的科研工作与清华大学合作，由崔福斋教授联合培养，博士论文《组织工程化骨修复兔下颌骨缺损同期种植体植入的实验研究》被中国口腔医学年鉴 2007 年卷优秀博士论文摘要栏目收入。2007 年 7 月，任锦州市中心医院眼、耳鼻喉、口腔教研室副主任；2010 年，遴选为辽宁医学院口腔系硕士研究生导师。2011 年，作为援疆干部赴新疆裕民，任裕民县卫生局副局长、县人民医院院长。现为辽宁医学院附属第二医院副院长。

攻读博士学位期间，在最初确定自己研究方向时充满着困惑，一时间难以找到科研道路的大门。通过查阅大量自己感兴趣的组织工程学方向的文献，并通过不断学习，了解到崔福斋教授是这方面的专家和国内外名副其实的权威，崔福斋教授长期从事生物材料科学与工程的研究，主要科研成就集中在骨、牙生物材料的机理研究以及生物材料表面改性等方面，取得多项开创性重大研究成果，在国际生物材料学界有着显著的影响。崔教授的出现，如这炉炭的殷红，给我无限温暖，带我走进了一个彩色的天地，一个充满无限希望和可能的科研世界。当时的我有如从朔风凛冽的户外来到冬日雪夜的炉边。

于是，我怀着无比激动和忐忑的心情，抱着试一试的态度，给崔老师发了邮件，令我意想不到的是，在我看来应当工作繁忙的崔老师却很快给我回信。这让我有些不知所措和难以相信。礼贤下士一直是中华民族的儒家文化中重要的价值观，但在我之前的求学生涯中却很少见到，也许是我已经习惯了老师们高高在上、学生诚惶诚恐的学习生活姿态。然而，崔老师给我的邮件回复中，并未见得任何居高临下的姿态，反而字里行间充满了无尽的关爱，体现身份差别的仅为长者之风。我不禁为这位老师所折服，原来站得高不仅望得远，还可以抬头正视前方。

崔老师严谨的科研态度和谦逊、朴素的为人处世之风已在回复我的邮件中给我留下了深刻的印象，更让我感到难以置信的是，作为一名国内外的知名学者竟主动提议让一个从未见面的我当面商议未来实验的研究方向。这位科研老人的平易近人令人折服。于是，便有了我第一次的清华求学之旅。同崔老师见面后更能切身体会到这位科研巨人的和蔼可亲。在崔福斋老师的指导下，我有针对性的认真学习了有关核心课程，为自己的科研工作打下扎实基础；并涉猎了一部分其他课程，开阔视野，对自己研究方向的应用背景以及整个学科的结构有了宏观的认识。

崔老师不仅学养深厚，而且谦虚谨慎，实事求是。从始至终，崔老师认真负责地给予我深刻而细致的指导，帮助我开拓研究思路，精心点拨，热忱鼓励。就这样，我在崔老师的指导帮助下发表了科研道路上的第一篇 SCI 文章。

花开花落，雁归雁去，时光就在不知不觉中匆匆流逝了。工作之后，我同崔老师建立起一种亦师亦友的深厚友谊，崔老师的为人处世、治学之道也对我成为研究生导师之后的工作产生了很大的影响。崔老师为人随和热情，治学严谨细心，敢于坚持真理，在学术观点上，既不人云亦云，亦不一味追求标新立异，充分体现了实事求是、求真务实的学者本色。同时，光明磊落地做人，诚挚热心地待人，公平、公正的为人处世的态度不仅为我树立了榜样，同样也深深地影响着我科研团队中的新生力量——硕士研究生。从他（她）们身上传递出的正能量正是汲取于崔老师这位科研学者身上的营养，也必将影响到更多的后继求学者。

因为您的一片爱心的灌溉，一番耕耘的辛劳，必然会有桃李的绚丽，科研稻麦的金黄。祝福崔老师未来的科研之路绿树常青，硕果累累。与此同时，我诚挚地希望在此前合作的基础上展开进一步的更深层次的合作，让我们彼此培育出的科研之花永不凋零，芬芳永存。

最后，祝愿崔老师工作顺利，身体健康。

# 3.15　可降解金属及表面改性研究之拙见

杨静馨

北京联合大学机电学院材料科学与工程系，北京

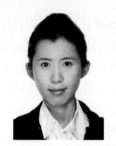

杨静馨，崔福斋教授 2006 级直博毕业生，博士培养时间：2006 年 9 月—2011 年 6 月。主要从事镁合金、钴铬合金等金属材料表面生物功能化改性研究，博士毕业论文题目是《镁合金和钴铬合金表面涂层的生物功能化研究》。博士期间在 SCI 收录期刊上作为第一作者共发表文章 9 篇。毕业后就职于航天科工集团第三研究院 8359 所，工程师。主要从事导弹发射系统设计工作。现任北京联合大学机电学院材料科学与工程系讲师。

　　从小学、中学、一路到大学，从来没停下来仔细想过未来做什么。做了这么多年的学生，即使到了本科结束，要读研究生，要读博士，真正要进入科研，依然觉得来得那么突然。一方面觉得一直处于理论的海洋中，没有实际应用，害怕自己驾驭不了；一方面科研好像玄而又玄，如何做？如何做得好？这些仿佛天天在头脑中纠缠。这个时候真真体会到"导师"这个词取得如此贴切。

　　崔老师是我研究生期间的导师，更是我的人生导师，从本科毕设到毕业前后 6 年，崔老师在学业、生活、工作等方面一直给予我很大的帮助，相比称呼崔教授，我更喜欢称呼崔老师，感觉更加亲切。崔老师更像一位长者，像父亲一般，如《鸣沙石室佚书——太公家教》里的"弟子事师，敬同于父，习其道也，学其言语。……忠臣无境外之交，弟子有束修之好。一日为师，终身为父。"崔老师就如同父亲一般，言传身教。

　　第一次发邮件，很快收到了崔老师的回信，约定了时间见面。第一次见崔老师是在他的办公室，平和的语气，直入主题的谈话，让我印象深刻。询问我的在校成绩，询问我的综合排名。之后立刻就让办公室的师兄带我去接触实验

室，我紧张到极致的神经瞬间放松下来。我每天在懵懂间，跟着师兄、师姐们做实验。比较顺利地完成了本科毕业设计，毕业论文被评为了优秀毕业论文。但是仿佛还是在跟循着足迹一般前进，找不到自己的方向。

突然有一天，崔老师叫我到办公室，有人参加国际会议回来，在跟崔老师讨论会议上的新的研究关注点。崔老师认为，镁合金作为首次考虑植入人体的可降解金属，具有极高的科研前景，必然会迅速发展，应用方面也会很广泛。崔老师说：目前这个方向德国公司走在最前[1]，国内还没有相关研究，在国际会议上也是第一次见报道。而且，我本科也是学金属材料的，希望我将精力投入到这上面，去调研国内外相关文献资料，了解研究动态，找到此方向的突破口，争取第一时间拿出好的结果，就能最快的发表高水平文章。崔老师直入主题，开始引导我寻找课题方向并选题。

2009 年冬天，经过一番调研，我找到了关键的突破口，就是研究组原有的仿生矿化基础，利用钙磷盐在带负电金属表面的沉积，在可降解镁合金表面首次利用仿生方法形成羟基磷灰石涂层，一方面提高了镁合金用于骨修复的生物相容性，一方面达到了人工调控镁合金降解速率的目的。这完全来自于组内原有的研究基础，在钛合金表面通过仿生法形成涂层，但当时只是想在金属表面得到一层矿化涂层。我后面的课题研究就依此慢慢展开，每一步前进都是利用了原有的研究基础，以一个临床上面的需求或者可能应用的闪光点为前提。这完全与本书的书名——《温故而知创新》吻合，这正是科研一步一步开展的重要基石。

我的第一篇文章让我真正体会到了发表文章的各种困难：换期刊投稿，一个期刊反复多次，每次很多而且复杂的评审意见，反复修改，补充实验，连续几周都是伴着早上射入窗帘的第一缕阳光小憩一会。印象最深刻，也是最生动的一个例子，就是当年过年回家的火车票因为修改文章，一而再，再而三的往后推。反复了一年，原本计划的尽快发表，也因此大大推迟了，虽然最后发表了[2]，现在回忆起来，耽误的时间仍旧是心中的一个挥之不去的伤痕。还好，之后的文章发表基本就一帆风顺了。可能这也是每个做科研的人都要经历的事情。

"生物可降解金属"的概念在 2006 年本身就是一个非常新的概念，尤其是在国内，逐渐在英文翻译上出现，但因为应用的目的不同，材料不同，尤其是文章写作者的理解不同，使用过诸如 biometal、bioabsorbable、biodegrable 等英文词汇来描述。本身生物材料就是一个高度融合的交叉学科，就我开始研究此课题的最初理解，我是从金属材料本身出发，所以更重视镁合金作为可降解金属的不足，就是降解速率过快的问题，所以我的文章中基本都是使用 biodegrable。此困惑一直存在，直到 2015 年 11 月参加 2015 全国生物材料大会，北京大学郑玉峰老师提到命名这个问题，经过多方求证，才使得 biodegrable metal

（BM）基本确定下来。

可降解金属材料是生物材料研究领域的一个热点，也是金属生物材料领域多方关注的问题。可降解金属是指在体内逐渐被腐蚀，有着较好的生物相容性，降解产物不会引起宿主反应，经过复杂过程，可以被人体慢慢吸收或者排出体外，没有植入物的残留的材料。从 2009 年开始，每年都会举行有关可降解金属的国际会议，这方面的研究数据大幅度增长。中国科学家在这个方面的研究做出了很大的贡献，就发表文章来看，重点有几个方面：新的可降解金属、可降解金属的微观结构、可降解金属的机械性能和体内外的降解行为。现在也有很多文章高屋建瓴地剖析可降解金属[3]。目前发展起来的主要的可降解金属有镁基、铁基、锌基 3 种，因为研究开展时间不同，镁基可降解金属材料已经进入临床阶段，研究最为深入。对于可降解金属以后的发展方向，集中在制备新的可降解金属体系、可降解金属的多孔结构、可降解金属的表面改性、新的制备方法等方面。

对于解决可降解金属的降解速率问题，从材料方面来说就有很多方法，我选择了表面改性。这也是后面我所有研究方向串联起来的一个关键研究问题。最开始的表面改性只是为了控制降解速率，后来逐步发展到调控表面机械性能，改善生物相容性功能，通过表面改性制备药物缓释系统等生物功能化的研究。表面改性的代表文章为 *Modification of degradation behavior of magnesium alloy by IBAD coating of calcium phosphate*，这篇文章的创新也出自组内的原有科研基础[4]，也是在温故过程中的一次创新。这篇文章是在调研金属表面改性方法时，结合本研究组内的优势，针对性比较强的一次尝试；是在前面镁合金基底制备仿生涂层后，结合力不好的情况下，针对提高结合力，使用了比较新颖的表面改性技术——离子束辅助沉积，而且创新地使用了钙磷涂层来调控降解速率。取得的实验结果非常满意，比较快地完成了文章写作，也很顺利地发表了文章。

毕业之前的博士论文撰写阶段，回顾自己的整个研究生的科研工作，研究课题比较分散，不同的材料，针对解决不同的问题，采用不同的表面改性方法，诸多方面，有深有浅。我自己总是在反复思考，如何完成自己的博士论文，需要数量，更需要质量，也就是既要有高度，也需要有深度。崔老师结合我几年的科研结果，给我指出了前面我提到过的主线：生物功能化的表面改性。这个题目几经周折才最终确定下来。

往往每一次的创新都需要一个灵感，这个灵感来自不停地汲取知识的过程，对于我，就是不停地去查阅文献，吸收文献精髓；参加会议，跟相关领域学者讨论。对于交叉学科，很关键的就是相互交流。很多时候，即使如前面的做到了，但往往高度不够，敏锐度不够，还是抓不到创新的那个关键点，这个时候去跟崔老师讨论一下，往往几分钟的收获胜过自己多日的琢磨。在我科研

的道路上，所做的创新都来自于崔老师的指点。举几个例子来结束我这部分的内容：

（1）讲文献。每个人的时间精力有限，不可能将所在领域的文献全部看过吸收。有一次组会前，崔老师给我一篇纸质文献，让我组会给大家讲讲。短短几十分钟，看完一篇英文文献，关键要吸收为自己的东西再给大家讲出来，任务完成得不好。但那次以后我发现，对文献的高效理解，是做创新极为关键的一步。创新不仅仅要讲究新，也要注重效率。一个新颖的创新点，设计好实验，得出结果，发表出来，时间过去，可能就不是创新了。

（2）国际会议。崔老师研究组的学生，基本每个人都有参加各种国际会议的经历。崔老师很看重学生的能力培养，让学生去做口头报告，我还被邀请做过邀请报告。经过这些，我觉得自己的综合能力得到了提升。会议过程中，除了多关注自己的方向，也要为同组其他方向做好记录，回到组里，要给大家讲参会的收获。往往会议的报道是最新的，这时的一句话、一个实验设计，可能都会给科研工作者很大的启发。

（3）交叉融合，相互学习。生物材料作为交叉学科，我们的课题往往就是多学科相互配合而完成的。制备的材料最终都是为了人体使用，因此，我们会经常与医院交流合作。材料领域科研人员每天埋头钻研，做出来的东西不实用，或者问题很多，在实验室我们永远发现不了，必须跟亲自使用的医生交流。我印象深刻的就是崔老师布置的一次任务，让我亲自去观摩手术，完成微小血管吻合器的设计。第一次身临其境的观摩手术，虽然之前做好了充分的思想准备，但还是不争气地晕在了手术室。不过，正是这次经历，使得微小血管吻合器的专利稿很顺利、很迅速地完成。

现在自己也在高校任教，对于科研的理解也有很多，但所有科研的思维、习惯等都是在研究生阶段形成的。以上都是自己研究生阶段的一点拙见，请批评指正。

## 培养期间代表性文章

1. Yang J X, Jiao Y P, Cui F Z, Lee I S, Yin Q S, Zhang Y. Modification of degradation behavior of magnesium alloy by IBAD coating of calcium phosphate. *Surface and Coatings Technology*, 2008, 202 (22-23): 5733-5736.

**Abstract**　In order to modify the degradation behavior of magnesium alloy, hydroxyapatite $[Ca_{10}(PO_4)_6(OH)_2]$ coating is formed on magnesium alloy by ion-beam assisted deposition (IBAD) and heat treatment. The morphology, composition and phase structure of the coated samples were investigated by scanning electron microscopy, energy dispersive X-ray spectroscopy, X-ray diffraction and Fourier trans-

form infrared spectroscopy, respectively. The width of atomic mixed interface between the coating and substrate formed by IBAD was approximate 3 μm, which was measured by Auger electron spectroscopy. The hardness and elastic modulus of coating were measured with a depth-sensing nanoindenter system. The results of accelerated test (AT) of degradation indicate that the coatings can decrease degradation rate of original Mg alloy significantly.

引用次数: **46**

2. Yang J X, Cui F Z, Lee I S. Surface Modifications of magnesium alloys for biomedical applications. *Annals of Biomedical Engineering*, 2011, 39 (7): 1857-1871.

**Abstract** In recent years, research on magnesium (Mg) alloys had increased significantly for hard tissue replacement and stent application due to their outstanding advantages. Firstly, Mg alloys have mechanical properties similar to bone which avoid stress shielding. Secondly, they are biocompatible essential to the human metabolism as a factor for many enzymes. In addition, main degradation product Mg is an essential trace element for human enzymes. The most important reason is they are perfectly biodegradable in the body fluid. However, extremely high degradation rate, resulting in too rapid loss of mechanical strength in chloride containing environments limits their applications. Engineered artificial biomaterials with appropriate mechanical properties, surface chemistry, and surface topography are in a great demand. As the interaction between the cells and tissues with biomaterials at the tissue-implant interface is a surface phenomenon; surface properties play a major role in determining both the biological response to implants and the material response to the physiological condition. Therefore, the ability to modify the surface properties while preserve the bulk properties is important, and surface modification to form a hard, biocompatible and corrosion resistant modified layer have always been an interesting topic in biomaterials field. In this article, attempts are made to give an overview of the current research and development status of surface modification technologies of Mg alloys for biomedical materials research. Further, the advantages/disadvantages of the different methods and with regard to the most promising method for Mg alloys are discussed. Finally, the scientific challenges are proposed based on own research and the work of other scientists.

引用次数: **38**

# 参考文献

[ 1 ]　Witte F, Fischer J, Nellesen J, et al. In vitro and in vivo corrosion measurements of mag-
　　　nesium alloys [J]. *Biomaterials*, 2006, 27 (7): 1013-1018.

[ 2 ]　Yang J X, Cui F Z, Jiao Y P, et al. Calcium phosphate coating on magnesium alloy for
　　　modification of degradation behavior [J]. *Frontiers of Materials Science in China*, 2008, 2
　　　(2): 143-148.

[ 3 ]　Hermawan H, Biodegradable metals: State of the art [J]. *Biodegradable Metals*, 2012:
　　　13-22.

[ 4 ]　Cui F Z, Luo Z S. Biomaterials modification by ion-beam processing [J]. *Surface and
　　　Coatings Technology*, 1999, 112 (1-3): 278-285.

# 3.16 科研中的"学"与"问"
## ——祝贺崔福斋教授 70 寿辰

刘 茜

耶鲁大学，美国

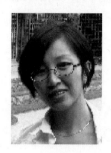

刘茜，2007 年，于清华大学材料科学与工程系攻读博士学位。2012 年毕业后在苏州大学工作，特聘副研究员。现在美国耶鲁大学从事博士后研究工作。

我于 2007 年年初加入崔老师的研究组，并于同年秋天在崔老师的指导下开始攻读博士学位。如同其他大多数博士生一样，我博士的第一年是在迷惘和纠结中度过的。崔老师耐心的帮助使我度过了这段艰难同时也是至关重要的时期，也让我渐渐明白了什么叫做学问，怎样去做研究。一个合格的科研工作者需要探索未知，拓宽人们的知识领域，并从中获得改善人们生活、提升社会价值的方法，最终造福整个人类。这是不可能一蹴而就的。

学问对于科研工作者而言，"学"的是已知的知识还有探索未知的方法，"问"的是未知，需要通过习得的探索方法去探求。所以通过学习文献来区别已知和未知是重中之重，这直接关系到所从事的研究工作有没有价值。崔老师十分重视这一点，时常要我们总结汇报国际前沿的科研动态，牢牢把握住已知、未知的分界线。正是基于这一点，我于 2009 年在崔老师的建议下开始从事干细胞和化学基团相互作用的研究。首先用真空沉积的办法在玻璃上镀一层金薄膜，然后利用硫醇单分子自组装的方法在金薄膜上构建高密度的特定化学基团。这种方法使得直接观察化学成分对干细胞的存活、迁移、分化的影响成为可能，加深了人们对于干细胞的理解，并进一步为优化干细胞疗法添砖加瓦。

如果说"学"决定了一个人的工作有没有价值，那么"问"则直接影响到他工作价值的高低。崔老师经常说：一个优秀的科研工作者可以用有限的资源解决重大的问题，而其中的关键就在于"问"。老实说，这个要求对于一个博士生来说太高了，一个博士生工作意义的大小很大程度上取决于他的导师。我本人很幸运地能够得到崔老师的指导，做出了真正意义上有价值的工作。生物医用材料服务于医疗，能够有效地治疗疾病，最大程度地缓解患者痛苦的材料就是好材料，相关的研究才是真正有价值的工作。然而，在我刚开始接手可注射骨修复材料的时候并不是这么想的，或者更坦率地说，我内心还是比较抗拒的。当初我觉得研究组里面对于骨修复材料的研究已经相当成熟了，至于材料是手术植入还是可注射在科学意义上又有什么区别呢？如今想来，当时的我起码想错了两点。首先，可注射骨修复材料适用于微创骨组织修复，更易于接触受损部位，在减少了患者痛苦的同时实现了更优化的治疗效果，因此，具有十分重大的应用意义。其次，一项研究的科学意义不是简简单单地看一看大概内容就能决定的。在从事这项课题研究的过程中，我发现仅仅是平衡材料的可注射性和机械支撑性能就需要考量胶体化学、非平衡态物理、生物矿化，还有实际的临床操作，是一个非常复杂的系统工程，具有很高的科学价值。

从博士入学的那一天开始，我从事科研工作已经 8 年多了，其中包括了在清华大学攻读博士的 5 年，在苏州大学工作的两年，直至眼下在耶鲁大学从事博士后研究，我深深地明白科研工作的不易。科学研究需要一个人全身心不计回报地投入，需要百折不挠的毅力，以及对知识、对真理的坚持和忠诚。70 岁的崔老师从事科研已逾 40 年，这份执着始终鼓励着我。韩愈说："师者，所以传道授业解惑也。"在指导我博士研究期间，崔老师一直牢牢地扮演了"传道"、"授业"和"解惑"的角色。然而，从更广的人生跨度来看，崔老师还是我人生的标杆和灯塔。当我自满时，可以拿来比一比，去掉心头的浮躁；当我迷惘时，可以拿来照一照，找到前行的目标。

谨以此文祝崔福斋老师 70 岁生日快乐。

## 培养期间代表性文章

Liu X, Wang X M, Horii A, Wang X J, Qiao L, Zhang S G, Cui F Z. In vivo studies on angiogenic activity of two designer self-assembling peptide scaffold hydrogels in the chicken embryo chorioallantoic membrane. *Nanoscale*, 2012, 4 (8): 2720-2727.

**Abstract** The rapid promotion of angiogenesis is critical for tissue engineering and regenerative medicine. The angiogenic activity of tissue-engineered scaffolds has already been the major criterion for choosing and designing ideal biological materials. We here report systematic in vivo studies on the angiogenic activity of two functionalized self-assembling peptides PRG ( Ac-( RADA )$_4$ GPRGDSGYRGDS-CONH$_2$ ) and KLT ( Ac-( RADA )$_4$ G$_4$ KLTWQELYQLKYKGI-CONH$_2$ ) using the chicken embryo chorioallantoic membrane ( CAM ) assay. 3D migration/sprouting bead assays showed that the two functional motifs PRGDSGYRGDS and KLTWQELYQLKYKGI improved the bioactivities of the self-assembling peptide RADA16-I ( Ac-( RADA )$_4$-CONH$_2$ ) dramatically and provided ideal synthetic microenvironments for endothelial cell migration and cordlike structure sprout formation. A CAM assay was carried out to assess the efficiency of various peptide scaffolds in inducing capillary invasion in vivo. Among these three peptide scaffolds, the functionalized peptide scaffold RAD/KLT presented a significantly better angiogenic activity inducing CAM tissue invasion and new capillary vessel formation within the scaffolds in the absence of VEGF. With the addition of VEGF, more newly formed vessel lumen could be observed in all peptide scaffolds. Our results suggested that the functionalized peptide scaffolds had satisfactory angiogenic properties, and may also have wide potential applications in tissue regeneration.

引用次数：**23**

# 3.17 干细胞及其共培养技术在骨组织工程中的应用
## ——祝贺崔老师 70 周岁生日

### 马金玲

#### 首都医科大学附属北京口腔医院，北京

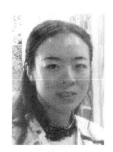 马金玲，2005 年，毕业于华北理工大学口腔医学系；2005—2008 年，于首都医科大学攻读口腔医学硕士学位；2008 年 11 月—2013 年，于荷兰奈梅亨大学攻读医学博士学位，并于 2013 年 11 月学成归国。2014 年 1 月至今，在首都医科大学附属北京口腔医院从事口腔种植等相关工作。博士课题研究方向为干细胞在骨组织工程中的应用。博士毕业论文题目为 *Cell-based strategies in bone tissue engineering：Effects of mesenchymal stem cell type and coculture with angiogenic cells*。共在 SCI 收录期刊上发表文章 15 篇，在国内核心期刊上发表文章 2 篇。曾多次在国内外重要学术会议上做口头演讲并担任大会主持。2015 年荣获"北京市优秀青年人才"荣誉称号。

    能够认识并成为崔福斋老师的学生是我人生中很幸运的事情。2007 年，正在首都医科大学读硕士研究生的我有幸认识崔老师，并在崔老师的指导下修改完成且在 *Journal of Tissue Engineering and Regenerative Medicine* 上发表我的硕士文章。这是我的第一篇 SCI 文章，作为首次接触英文文章写作的我来说，是一次挑战，也进步很大，这得益于崔老师的悉心指导和教诲。之后的一年里，我所在的潘巨利教授的研究组与崔老师的研究组交流合作频繁，我也经常参加师弟、师妹们的课题讨论，参与课题设计，多次参加崔老师课题组的交流讨论。期间，有共鸣，有火花，当然也有争议，也正因为这些，让我更加领悟了科研的真正含义，从懵懂到清晰。同时，也更加领略了崔老师在学术方面的严谨、执着和前瞻性。

    2008 年，在我硕士毕业前夕，在崔老师的引荐下，我有幸得到了一个参

加中荷合作项目并开始长达近5年的荷兰博士留学生涯的机会。当时被告知要做的研究方向是骨组织工程和生物材料，对于我一个医学背景的人来讲，对组织工程略知一二已经很不错了，对生物材料就更加陌生，尤其是生物材料的基础和机理部分。这时，崔老师给了我一个学习的好机会，在出国前短短的几个月内，在他的实验室参观学习并参加材料科学与工程系课程的学习。崔老师也会隔三差五给我讲解生物材料课程的奥秘。这段时间，每天奔波于逸夫技术科学楼与教学楼之间，体会着清华学生的快节奏和良好的学习氛围，被周围的每一个人感染着。可以说，清华大学短短几个月的交流学习为我出国深造打下了很好的基础，也是一个良好的开端，是一笔人生难得的财富和体验。同时，也感谢崔老师在这段日子里对我的启蒙和帮助。

2008年11月，我正式开始了为期近5年的荷兰留学生活。刚到荷兰的日子里，有些许不适应，毕竟是只身一人，而且是异国他乡。记得每每跟崔老师打电话报平安，崔老师都会给我鼓劲并告诉我他当年在荷兰的生活、工作经历和经验。很快地，生活、工作都步入了正轨。在荷兰做科研期间，我经常与崔老师交流我的课题设计，他都会毫无保留地给我提出宝贵的意见与建议，中肯而有价值。我每次回国都会去拜访崔老师，跟他探讨我的课题，聊聊荷兰的生活。崔老师也会很自豪地跟我聊他们研究组获得国家自然科学奖的事情，或是他作为杰出代表被国家领导人接见的场景。就这样，我的留学生活一直有条不紊地进行着，并于2013年11月顺利获得荷兰博士学位并回国。

荷兰留学期间的研究方向是干细胞技术在骨组织工程中的应用。毕业论文题目是 *Cell-based strategies in bone tissue engineering : effects of mesenchymal stem cell type and coculture with angiogenic cells*。围绕干细胞的单培养或共培养两种手段，应用不同种类的干细胞，实现骨组织工程的成功。同时，共培养技术，也即将干细胞与血管内皮细胞一起培养，可以实现骨组织工程中的血管化。荷兰留学的几年，是自己知识积累快速提升的几年，同时，也是不断汲取新知识和学习新技术的几年，更是自己科研的逻辑思维不断完善和提高的几年。在此期间，我很幸运地参加了几次国际学术交流大会。而且，在维也纳的第3届世界骨组织工程和再生医学大会上有幸担任大会主持。可以说，我无悔于荷兰的留学生涯，相反，我很庆幸自己当初选择了留学。再次感谢崔老师对我荷兰留学的推荐、帮助与鼓励！

2014年1月至今，我在首都医科大学附属北京口腔医院特诊特需科工作。作为一名种植医生，我深知病人缺牙和种植区骨量不足的痛苦，也领悟到骨组织工程应用于临床的紧迫性和重要性。崔老师的研究组有着坚实的科研基础和强大的科研团队，在科研的构思、设计、实施等方面都可信、可靠。希望未来的日子里，我能与崔老师的研究组有更加深入的交流与合作。

# 培养期间代表性文章

Ma J L, van den Beucken J JJP, Yang F, Both S K, Cui F Z, Pan J L, Jansen J A. Coculture of osteoblasts and endothelial cells: Optimization of culture medium and cell ratio. *Tissue Engineering Part C: Methods*, 2010, 17 (3): 349-357.

**Abstract** Vascularization strategies in cell-based bone tissue engineering depend on optimal culture conditions. The present study aimed to determine optimal cell culture medium and cell ratio for cocultures of human marrow stromal cells (HMSCs) and human umbilical vein endothelial cells (HUVECs) in view of both osteogenic and angiogenic outcome parameters upon two-dimensional and three-dimensional culture conditions. Cultures were performed in four different media: osteoblastic cell proliferation medium, osteogenic medium (OM), endothelial medium, and a 1 : 1 mixture of the latter two media. Mineralization within the cocultures was observed only in OM. Subsequent experiments in OM showed that alkaline phosphatase activity, mineralization, and CD31 (+) staining were highest for cocultures at a 50 : 50 HMSC/HUVEC ratio. Therefore, the results from the present study show that a HMSC/HUVEC coculture ratio of 50 : 50 in OM is the best combination to obtain both osteogenic and angiogenic differentiation.

引用次数: **24**

# 3.18　崔福斋教授和他的骨材料

## 俞　兴

北京中医药大学东直门医院，北京

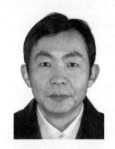

俞兴，主任医师，博士生导师。分别于 1995 年和 2002 年获得北京大学医学部临床医学学士、博士学位；2002—2004 年，于清华大学材料科学与工程系生物材料组从事博士后研究工作，合作导师为崔福斋教授，首次将纳米人工骨应用于临床，被评为清华大学特优博士后。现任北京中医药大学东直门医院骨科Ⅲ主任、脊柱脊髓专业组组长。兼任中国康复医学会骨与关节及风湿病专业委员会常务务员及常务秘书、中国残疾人康复医学会脊柱脊髓损伤专业委员会常务委员、中国康复医学会脊柱非融合学组委员及秘书、中国康复医学会术中影像和骨科导航学组常务委员和秘书、中国生物材料学会骨修复材料与器械分会委员、中国医师协会骨科分会骨科康复工作委员会委员。《生物骨科材料与临床研究》特约编委，《中华现代外科杂志》常务编委，《中国组织工程研究与临床康复杂志》常务编委、专家库成员，《生物医学工程与临床杂志》编委。

初识崔福斋教授清晰如昨日，细一想已是 10 余年前的事。

博士毕业那年，因为一些原因，不能继续留在自己学习、工作的北京大学人民医院，经人介绍和引荐准备到崔福斋教授的生物材料实验室做博士后。那是 2002 年夏天的一个傍晚，下午 4 点，我如约敲开了清华大学逸夫科学技术楼崔教授办公室的门，没等我开口说话，崔教授用带着南方口音的普通话像熟人相见似的说道："俞兴，坐吧，这是我的两位博士，研究方向一个是骨材料、一个是神经材料，与你的研究有互补，今后你们之间沟通的机会会很多。"随后，崔教授介绍了生物材料实验室的研究重点和方向，两位博士各自介绍了自己的研究内容，我也介绍了博士期间的工作。你一言我一语，谈话进行得很融洽，离开崔教授办公室已是两小时以后。崔教授对医学知识的了解，尤其是对人体骨微结构的研究，让我这个骨科博士都自叹不如。十几年过去了，那天的谈话仍记忆犹新，因为正是那天与崔教授的谈话让我下定决心到清华大学做博士后，而在清华大学做博士后的这短短两年是我骨科生涯中成长最快、收获最丰的时期，而这些都得感谢崔福斋教授。

那时崔老师（我们学生更喜欢用崔老师这个称呼，哪怕是在多年以后）及其研究团队研发的纳米晶胶原基骨材料在实验室已历时近 10 年，他们从研究胚胎骨的发生、骨折愈合、骨痂转归过程入手，深入探索骨的形成构建机制。在此基础上，利用生物自组装原理在常温下合成了微结构接近人体松质骨的人工骨，成分和结构双重仿生，这是传统陶瓷人工骨不可能实现的，因为陶瓷人工骨需高温烧结，而高温将破坏胶原的活性。这在当时是一大突破，而且研究结果具有国人的自主知识产权，因此，在国内外骨材料研发领域引起了巨大反响。但骨材料的研发不同于其他材料，它最终的目的是获得临床应用并被临床认可，走出实验室、走进临床才是这近 10 年研究的目的，崔老师心底非常清楚下一步的努力方向。但实验室的研究成果如何才能走出实验室、走进临床，其困难和艰巨性是可想而知的。清华大学许多以往材料方面的研究课题，文章、专利不少，但都没有实际应用，最后绝大部分研究成果只能躺在实验室里不了了之。崔老师最不愿自己倾尽全力研发的骨材料也是此结果，让研发多年的骨材料造福于临床患者才是他最大的心愿。为此崔老师不断与企业、骨科医生、质检机构交流联系。隔行如隔山，崔老师虽然已是清华大学材料科学与工程系生物材料实验室的首席科学家，但他对骨科临床要求、产品审批流程等方面的知识了解不多，为了更好地与其他领域的专家沟通，他不断查阅、研究骨材料获得临床审批所需的每一个环节，不断学习骨科临床对骨材料需求的适用范围，不断去完善基础研究和补充申报材料，此过程每前进一步均要付出大量的精力（而这些精力的付出不同于实验室的研究，除执着以外，更需要丰富的社会经验的沉淀，这也是清华大学大部分研究型教授所缺乏且不屑去做的，也是他们研究成果沉睡的一个主要原因）。这么多年，我目睹了崔老师在这一方面从零的起步到成为目前国内为数不多的产学研一体化的资深专家、行业领航人，而这其中的艰辛、困惑和无奈，我想只有他自己本人才清楚，不是我们做学生的三言两语所能描述的。

2002 年 11 月 27 日是一个特殊的日子，经过崔老师及其合作企业数年的不懈努力，终于在这一天纳米晶胶原基骨材料获得临床试验许可。虽然仅是一个临床试验许可，但崔老师非常清楚这个许可的重要性，有了这个许可，研发多年的骨材料才能用于临床骨缺损的修复，而只有临床证实了此骨材料修复骨缺损的效果，此骨材料才有可能成为骨修复产品，去造福广大的临床患者。现在我依然记得崔老师打电话告诉我这个消息时的激动，"俞兴，我们的骨材料临床试验许可下来了，下面就等你去找第一例患者了！"接到电话的这一刻我正在北京大学人民医院的动物房，在大鼠胫骨骨缺损模型上验证我们骨材料的安全性和修复效果。虽然在我做博士后之前，已有多个动物实验证实了此骨材料的安全性和骨修复效果，但因为不是自己亲自做的实验，我对所得的实验数据仍不放心，在用到患者体内之前，我最好能自己重复部分动物实验。当时，还担心崔老师不同意这种重复性的动物实验，不想崔老师对我的想法很是支持，爽快地答应了。所以 8 月份进站后，我大部分时间都在动物房、放射科和病理切片室。3 个多月 30 只大鼠的实验结果以及动物实验之余对此骨材料研发所有相关文献的恶补打消了我心底对此骨材料临床应用的顾虑和担忧。因此，当我接到崔老师的电话时，回答非常干脆，"崔老师，我来找第一个患者！"在以后 1 年半的时间内，我完成了《纳米晶胶原基骨材料的临床初步研究》的博士后出站报告，完成了 100 余例临床试验，并被评为清华大学特优博士后。现在回想起来，自己只不过做了一个骨科医生和研究者应做的事，重要的是崔老师的各方面努力才使我有机会在临床上率先应用纳米晶胶原基骨材料。《中国医学论坛报》将"纳米晶胶原基骨材料临床应用"评为 2003 年医学十大新闻之一，足见当年的影响之大。

崔老师虽然是我的博士后合作导师，但我平时大部分时间都用在临床，每周回实验室 1~2 次，也是来也匆匆去亦匆匆，查完资料就走，专门见崔老师的机会很少，即使相见，崔老师对我也很客气，把我当做合作的骨科医生看待。崔老师对学生的严格要求是在我参加组会时才见证的，并给我留下深刻印象。研究组定时召开组会，让学生汇报近期研究进展，组会我一般都争取参加，一方面了解组里博士、硕士的研究动向，另一方面有时我从医学角度提点自己的建议，生物材料的研究常涉及多个学科的交叉，不同研究背景的人在一起讨论，能扩大各自的视野。组会时，崔老师让与会学生逐一汇报，他要求每人汇报的思路必须清晰、重点突出，而他的点评更是简洁干脆，常一语中的，对不满意之处的批评从不留情面，有时甚至有点让人下不了台。现在偶尔有机会与那时的博士、硕士相遇，提起那段时间的研究经历，他们常常感慨，如果没有崔老师当时的严格要求，也不会有如今在各自领域上的成绩。2014 年这一年，崔老师有 3 个学生在不同的高校同时评为教授，崔老师说起此事，言语间充满了幸福感，丝毫没有当年不苟言笑、严厉批评的痕迹。

博士后出站后，与崔老师的合作关系一直延续至今，虽然见面机会不多，但对崔老师的研发一直很关注。每次相见，谈起骨材料的研发，都能从崔老师的言语中收获他的新思维、新想法。而且觉得崔老师一次比一次年轻、精神好，向崔老师询问其中秘诀，崔老师总是笑而不答，其实学生心底有数：不为名利所累，做自己喜欢之事，心态释然，人自然年轻。值老师古稀之际，以文忆点滴，共贺之。

# 培养期间代表性文章

Yu X, Xu L, Zhang X D, Cui F Z. Effect of spinal cord injury on urinary bladder spinal neural pathway: A retrograde transneuronal tracing study with pseudorabies virus. *Urology*, 2003, 62 (4): 755-759.

**Abstract**  Objectives. To determinate the effect of acute and chronic spinal cord injury (SCI) resulting from thoracic cord transection on the urinary bladder spinal neural pathway.

Methods. Seventy-six adult Sprague-Dawley rats were randomly divided into four groups, non-SCI (normal rats undergoing no surgical procedure except pseudorabies virus [PRV] injection), $SCI_b$ (SCI and PRV injected immediately after SCI), $SCI_c$ (SCI and PRV injected at 3 weeks after SCI), and $SCI_d$ (SCI and PRV injected at 3 months after SCI). Transcardiac perfusion fixation was done at appropriate survival periods after PRV injection into the bladder wall tissue. Sections of the dorsal root ganglion, spinal cord, and brain were processed for visualization of the virus by the streptavidin-peroxidase immunohistochemical procedure.

Results. The bladder weight of the non-SCI, $SCI_b$, $SCI_c$, $SCI_d$ rats was $144\pm9$ mg, $142\pm8$ mg, $486\pm51$ mg, and $656\pm69$ mg, respectively. The time-ordered flow charts of PRV tracing were similar in the non-SCI and SCI rats. The cross-sectional area of the labeled dorsal root ganglion cell profiles increased significantly after SCI ($P < 0.001$): $593\pm40$ $\mu m^2$, $588\pm39$ $\mu m^2$, $815\pm53$ $\mu m^2$, and $902\pm57$ $\mu m^2$ in the non-SCI, $SCI_b$, $SCI_c$, $SCI_d$ rats, respectively. The number of labeled cells in the dorsal horn in the L6 and S1 segments 3 days after PRV injection markedly increased in chronic SCI rats, as did the number of labeled motor neurons 4 days after injection.

Conclusions. Acute and chronic SCI have no effect on the process of virus transneuronal transport below the level of the lesion. Subsequent to chronic SCI, reorganization of the micturition reflex pathways may occur.

引用次数：**11**

# 3.19　表面改性：生物材料的热点话题

焦延鹏

暨南大学理工学院材料科学与工程系，广州

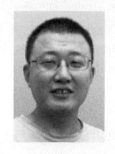

焦延鹏，暨南大学理工学院材料科学与工程系研究员，博士生导师。2006年7月—2008年6月，在清华大学材料科学与工程系生物材料实验室从事博士后研究工作，合作导师为崔福斋教授。博士后期间主要从事镁合金材料的表面改性以及电纺丝血管组织工程支架的研究工作。2008年7月至今，在暨南大学理工学院材料科学与工程系工作。人工器官及材料教育部工程中心和广东省教育厅生物材料重点实验室的骨干成员。一直从事组织工程支架材料、医用抗菌材料以及药物载体材料的研究与开发，工作重点集中在材料的表面改性及其生物相容性研究。

　　2006年7月，从暨南大学的生物医学工程专业博士毕业，我有幸进入清华大学材料科学与工程系崔福斋老师的研究组继续从事博士后研究工作。在崔老师研究组工作的两年时间里，崔老师严谨求实的工作态度和渊博的知识体系对我后续所从事科研工作的影响非常大，培养了我积极、踏实的工作态度，也使我独立开展科研工作的能力得到很大的提升。在崔老师的指导下，博士后期间主要从事生物材料表面改性相关的研究工作，在我博士论文研究的基础上，大大拓宽了我在该领域研究的深度和广度，为我后续独立从事科研工作打下了基础。博士后期间，和崔老师合作发表了多篇研究文章，其中 *Surface modification of polyester biomaterials for tissue engineering* 目前的引用已经超过 130 次（Google Scholar）。

　　这篇文章以生物材料领域的一类明星材料——可降解的聚酯类材料为对象，较为系统地总结了这类材料的表面改性及其在组织工程中的应用。应该说，表面改性是生物材料领域一个永恒的话题，无论是血液相容性材料、医用金属材料、组织工程支架材料，还是生物纳米材料，表面改性在这些相关的研究中都扮演了重要的角色。对生物材料进行表面修饰，主要目的是在不改变材料的本体性能的基础上，使其与生物（大）分子、细胞和组织之间产生我们所期望的响应性。生物体内的表面化学的一个重要特征是高度的动态变化，因此，在制备生物材料时，必须考虑后续的血清（组织液）蛋白的吸附、细胞的黏附和迁移、细胞外基质的沉积和组织的重建等。在某种程度上讲，材料的初始性能，尤其是生物材料的表面性能，在生物材料功能性体现方面变得非常重要。接下来，就从几个方面来谈一下本人对生物材料表面改性的认识。

### 1. 医用金属材料

医用金属材料是目前临床上使用最多、发展最为成熟的一类生物材料，其主要特点是具有非常优异的力学性能。其中的人工关节、牙种植体和脊柱融合器这 3 类材料对表面性能的要求是非常高的，这些材料的一个共同的特点是需要材料的表面和骨组织之间具有良好的结合能力。目前，相当多的研究和开发是通过表面拓扑形貌的改变，通过有机/无机涂层技术来提高其与骨组织的亲和性，其中最具有代表性的是羟基磷灰石涂层技术。金属冠脉血管支架是另一类应用较为广泛的金属材料，虽然这类材料的研发方向是可降解，但是目前金属类材料仍然是临床应用的主流。这类材料研究的热点依然是表面改性，其主要的目的包括两大类：快速的内皮化和抗狭窄。前者主要是通过在材料表面引入与内皮化相关的功能性的分子（Arg-Gly-Asp 分子为代表）或可以捕获内皮祖细胞的分子（CD34 分子为代表）来实现，后者主要是通过药物（紫杉醇和雷帕霉素为代表）涂层技术，形成可洗脱的药物冠脉支架。

### 2. 组织工程支架材料

组织工程支架材料以及组织修复材料的发展，是基于对天然的细胞外基质结构的认识和理解。组织工程支架材料的制备主要基于 3 个尺寸范围：毫米或厘米尺度的宏观结构决定了工程化组织的形状和大小；微米尺度的孔径大小可以调节细胞或组织的长入和营养物质的交换；纳米尺度的表面性能则控制着细胞的黏附和基因表达。随着 3D 打印技术的快速发展，个性化地制备毫米和微米尺度的形状已经越来越成熟，尤其是该技术的发展使多组织的器官构建成为可能。目前，该领域的研究热点依然集中在纳米尺度和生物仿生的表面性能上，主要是通过调控材料表面的刚性，在材料表面引入特异性的结合位点（整合素特异性结合受体），实现其对所吸附蛋白的构象以及（干）细胞活性的调控，最终实现体外组织的构建，或者在体内实现对目标组织的诱导和最终修复。

### 3. 血液相容性材料

大部分的生物材料通常都会和血液系统接触，因此，良好的血液相容性也是生物材料的基本要求之一。其中人工血管、心脏封堵器是直接与血液接触来发挥作用。另外，一些生物纳米材料是通过静脉注射的方式来实现其治疗和诊断的目的，这些材料会与血液中复杂的组分（血浆蛋白、补体系统、红细胞、白细胞和血小板等）发生复杂的相互作用，产生溶血、凝血以及补体激活等免疫相关的一系列反应。对于前者，在材料表面引入钝化层（PEG 为代表），减少与血液组分的接触可以实现良好的抗凝血性能。表面快速内皮化是目前研究的热点，在材料表面引入特异性分子，快速地从血液中捕获内皮祖细胞，最终实现内皮化。对于后者，除了尺寸的控制，在表面引入钝化层，减少材料对血液蛋白和细胞的作用是目前常用的方法。

4. 生物纳米材料

在生物材料研究中，药物/基因载体、分子影像造影剂以及免疫佐剂等生物纳米材料是重要的研究方向。这类材料得已临床应用的一个基本前提是体内（血液）的长效性、靶向性及细胞（核）穿透性。为了实现这 3 个目标，目前的研究主要也是围绕纳米材料的表面改性来进行的。为了实现体内的长效性，通常是将一些 PEG 类的材料连接到材料的表面，从而形成一层水化层，减少纳米材料表面蛋白的吸附和构象的变化，从而逃避机体免疫系统的捕获。为了实现纳米材料在靶位点（病变或癌变组织）的富集，通常是将一些靶位点细胞高表达受体的相应配体引入到纳米材料的表面，通过类似抗原-抗体的特异性结合，实现材料在靶位点的富集。经典的配体分子是叶酸和转铁蛋白体系。纳米基因载体和一些需要细胞内给药的纳米材料还要具有良好的细胞膜或/和核膜的穿透性，研究较多的是将一些疏水性的（核）膜穿透多肽引入到材料表面，最终实现细胞内或核内释药（基因）。

总之，从生物材料研发的初期到目前，乃至将来，生物材料的表面改性的研究一直是生物材料领域的一个热门研究领域。随着表面改性和表征技术的发展，以及人们对生物相容性的深入认识，表面改性依然会在该领域得到持续的发展。

# 培养期间代表性文章

Jiao Y P, Cui F Z. Surface modification of polyester biomaterials for tissue engineering. *Biomedical Materials*, 2007, 2（4）: R24-R37.

**Abstract** Surfaces play an important role in a biological system for most biological reactions occurring at surfaces and interfaces. The development of biomaterials for tissue engineering is to create perfect surfaces which can provoke specific cellular responses and direct new tissue regeneration. The improvement in biocompatibility of biomaterials for tissue engineering by directed surface modification is an important contribution to biomaterials development. Among many biomaterials used for tissue engineering, polyesters have been well documented for their excellent biodegradability, biocompatibility and nontoxicity. However, poor hydrophilicity and the lack of natural recognition sites on the surface of polyesters have greatly limited their further application in the tissue engineering field. Therefore, how to introduce functional groups or molecules to polyester surfaces, which ideally adjust cell/tissue biological functions, becomes more and more important. In this review, recent advances in polyester surface modification and their applications are reviewed. The development of new technologies or methods used to modify polyester surfaces for developing their biocompatibility is introduced. The results of polyester surface modifications by surface morphological modification, surface chemical group/charge modification, surface biomacromolecule modification and so on are reported in detail. Modified surface properties of polyesters directly related to in vitro/vivo biological performances are presented as well, such as protein adsorption, cell attachment and growth and tissue response. Lastly, the prospect of polyester surface modification is discussed, especially the current conception of biomimetic and molecular recognition.

引用次数：**84**

# 3.20  勇为人先，不断创新
## ——致礼崔福斋教授70寿辰

### 王 颖

首都医科大学基础医学院，北京

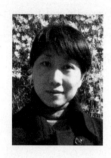

王颖，毕业于首都医科大学，2012年进入崔福斋教授生物材料研究组从事博士后研究，涉及多种生物材料和医学交叉学科相关研究，主要包括材料表面化学性状对神经干细胞的调控以及多肽水凝胶对中枢神经损伤的修复作用等。现就职于首都医科大学基础医学院，从事组织工程和干细胞技术在神经科学领域的应用研究。

我是崔福斋教授的博士后，主要做生物材料在中枢神经系统修复领域的开发应用以及作用机制方面的研究。在博士后工作几年中，领略了崔老师的风采，得到他的悉心指点，令我终身受益。谨以此文记录这一段珍贵而难忘的日子，献给崔老师70寿辰。

初识崔老师，你总会被他风风火火的行事风格吸引，就像一部高效运转而又精密控制的机器，思维敏捷，处事果断、迅速而井井有条，那排得满满的日程表就是他的写照。你也总会对他迅捷而跃动的思维、精深而广博的知识赞叹不已，看似千头万绪、杂乱无章的信息，他总能如抽丝剥茧、拨云见日般抓住问题核心，在不同学科间游刃有余。最重要的是他那对科学问题的把握，精准而超前，使得他总能走在科学研究的前沿。

众所周知，崔老师在骨组织工程材料研发领域早有建树，为我国自主骨修复材料的研发和推广、应用做出了巨大贡献。不仅如此，在中枢神经系统损伤修复方面，崔老师也是一位先行者，他与著名神经科学家、首都医科大学徐群渊教授研究组合作，开创性地将生物材料的应用引入这一领域。中枢神经系统作为机体的高级中枢，构造最为复杂，大量神经细胞有机地整合在一起构成复杂网络和回路，功能极其重要，控制了机体的生物行为，一旦损伤，自身难以修复，往往会造成伤残等非常严重的后果，给病人造成巨大痛苦，给家庭和社会带来巨大负担，目前，临床并无有效治疗方法。

虽然采用组织工程技术修复组织损伤已发展多年，但在脑和脊髓领域应用还是一片禁区，崔老师带领团队利用存在于细胞外基质的天然生物材料，合成了模拟中枢神经系统细胞外基质框架结构的水凝胶，并将水凝胶开创性地用于脑损伤修复研究，取得了可喜的效果。我有幸在神经修复团队中做了一部分工作，崔老师灵动的思维给我很多启发，他对关键科学问题的把握让研究方向始终朝着正确方向，对研究课题的高瞻远瞩也给我莫大的信心。想到早年在做博士后期间工作汇报时还有人指出这是异想天开的，甚至是难以接受的，可见，当时这一研究领域是多么超前。在这一领域中，崔老师团队的研究走到了最前列，从生物材料的筛选、合成、生物修饰，到神经干细胞的调控，直至动物体内组织水平的整体修复，从基础应用到机制研究系统，研究工作步步深入，发表了 10 余篇有影响力的科研文章。而今，国际上神经系统组织工程研究工作开展得如火如荼，备受瞩目。越来越多的医生、学者认识到干细胞和组织工程技术可能成为突破神经修复障碍的最有力工具。尤其可喜的是，国家也将其作为重点科研项目给予大力支持。在这项工作中，崔老师给我们带来了头脑风暴般的想法，我们也深刻体会到了创新的重要性，创新就是研究的生命，创新需要深厚的积累，创新更需要勇气。

借崔老师 70 寿辰之大喜，展望神经组织生物材料研究美好的未来，希望在崔老师的指引下，继续开创，深入研究，同时做好研究成果的转化工作，盼组织工程材料能早日为神经损伤的临床治疗带来福音，解除千千万万患者的病痛。

在此，衷心感谢敬爱的崔老师的引领和指导，感谢崔老师及其夫人的关怀和鼓励，感谢崔老师的榜样力量！愿崔老师身体健康，永远龙马精神！祝您 70 岁生日快乐吉祥！

# 培养期间代表性文章

Wang Y, Wei Y T, Zu Z H, Ju R K, Guo M Y, Wang X M, Xu Q Y, Cui F Z. Combination of hyaluronic acid hydrogel scaffold and PLGA microspheres for supporting survival of neural stem cells. *Pharmaceutical Research*, 2011, 28 （6）: 1406-1414.

**Abstract** Purpose. To develop a biomaterial composite for promoting proliferation and migration of neural stem cells （NSCs）, as well as angiogenesis on the materials, to rescue central nervous system （CNS） injuries.

Methods. A delivery system was constructed based on crosslinked hyaluronic acid （HA） hydrogels, containing embedded BDNF and VEGF-loaded poly （lactic-co-glycolic acid) (PLGA) microspheres for controlled delivery and support for NSCs in the CNS. The surface morphologies were evaluated by SEM and AFM, mechanical property was investigated by rheological tests, and release kinetics were performed by ELISA. Bioactivity of released BDNF and VEGF was assessed by neuron and endothelial cell culture, respectively. Compatibility with NSCs was studied by immunofluorescent staining.

Results. Release kinetics showed the delivery of BDNF and VEGF from PLGA microspheres and HA hydrogel composite were sustainable and stable, releasing ~20-30% within 150 h. The bioactivities preserved well to promote survival and growth of the cells. Evaluation of structure and mechanical properties showed the hydrogel composite possessed an elastic scaffold structure. Biocompatibility assay showed NSCs adhered and proliferated well on the hydrogel.

Conclusions. Our created HA hydrogel/PLGA microsphere systems have a good potential for controlled delivery of varied biofactors and supporting NSCs for brain repair and implantation.

引用次数: 34

# 3.21 画 龙 点 睛
## ——回顾我的博士后研究经历，以此谨祝崔福斋老师 70 岁生日

陈宗刚

山东大学，济南

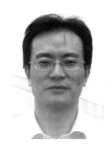

陈宗刚，1995 年，毕业于天津工业大学，后进入山东泰山制丝有限公司工作；2001 年，在天津工业大学材料科学与化学工程学院攻读硕士学位；2004 年毕业后，在东华大学攻读博士学位；2006 年 6 月—9 月，赴新加坡国立大学工程学院生物工程系进行合作研究；2008 年 3 月获得博士学位后，进入清华大学材料科学与工程系从事博士后研究，研究课题是可注射的骨修复材料。2010 年 10 月，进入山东大学国家糖工程技术研究中心，从事糖相关的生物材料研究工作。

众所周知，"画龙点睛"是比喻说话或做事时关键部位处理得好，使整体效果更加传神。回顾自己的学习生涯，感觉自己在清华大学跟随崔福斋先生进行博士后研究的经历，本身就是自己在学习、成长道路上的一处点睛之笔。在博士后研究过程中，得到先生许多的言传身教，在我看来也都是醍醐灌顶、画龙点睛。

我从读博士开始踏入生物材料研究领域，自从徜徉于生物材料的海洋，即闻先生在骨修复材料领域的声名和成就。在一次有关生物材料的学术"盛宴"上，终于得见先生真人和他的纳米晶矿化胶原基骨修复材料。怀着对生物材料研究的向往和对先生的崇敬，博士毕业后，我顺利地来到清华大学跟随先生进行我的博士后研究工作。

1. 做科研首先是做人

做科研首先是踏踏实实做人，勤勤恳恳做事，将学术当做毕生事业。这是我来到清华大学先生的实验室之后，先生以身作则首先给我的无言教诲。在他看来，做学问是很崇高而且能够给人带来极大快乐的事情。这样一种境界，对于我从事科研保持平和奋进的心态无疑是一种潜移默化的影响。科学研究和人

生的道路一样，不可能都是一路花雨。无论是在人生还是科研的旅途中，可能既有艳阳高照，也有阴霾满天，甚至是狂风暴雨。我们既要学会珍惜努力得来的顺境，又要经得起逆境的考验。自古以来，大凡有所成就者都要经历许多逆境的考验。人生不如意的事十有八九，如果总是怨天尤人，不会成为一个有出息的人。我不是一个有天赋的人，比较相信努力、相信付出才有收获。中国古训："业精于勤荒于嬉"。我深刻体会到要学会在喧闹中默默坚守，集中精力与目标，保持一颗坦荡的心，谦虚谨慎，戒骄戒躁，相信自己的努力可以产生巨大的能量，做好自己想做的事情。这是先生的言传身教带给我的人生感悟和启发。

### 2. 立足于应用做研究

先生做研究最得意之作应该就是他的纳米晶矿化胶原基骨修复材料，目前，在临床已经应用 10 多万例，因为这个研究成果为人类健康和社会发展做出的贡献，在 *Science* 上，先生被作为对中国组织工程研究做出突出贡献的人进行报道。因此，也可以看出先生对研究最终要为应用服务的立场。也正基于此，在我刚到清华大学，开始博士后课题研究之前，先生就让我先到他科研成果转化的孵化基地去实践调研。在那儿，我不但更详细地了解了科学研究向实际应用转化的过程，而且更激发了我对科学研究的兴趣和向往。在此基础上，先生提出想让我在纳米晶矿化胶原基骨修复材料的基础上研究可注射的骨修复材料。以便通过微创外科技术，在组织损伤小、不破坏修复区血供、操作简单易行、极大减轻病人痛苦的情况下修复骨组织创伤。复杂问题简单化，用半水硫酸钙作为注射载体和固化剂，与纳米晶矿化胶原基骨修复材料复合，利用半水硫酸钙良好的可注射性、自固化性能和矿化胶原基骨修复材料的良好成骨性，研发可注射骨修复材料。

半水硫酸钙和矿化胶原基骨修复材料都是已经临床应用的材料，复合开发可注射骨修复材料看似应该很容易解决。但是，两种材料混合并不一定代表两种材料性能的完全融合。在实施的过程中，也会遇到许多意想不到的麻烦。例如，材料固化成型后会发生溃散，力学性能不能满足要求，尤其是两种材料混合后，固化时间大幅度增加，不能适应临床需要等。科研中遇到困难，很容易让人产生烦躁情绪。这时，先生的谆谆教诲就会回响于心间：要善于吸取失败的教训，在实验中发现问题，勤于思考，找出失败的原因，提出克服失败的措施，才能最终取得成功。于是，摆正心态，重复实验，找出解决问题的方法和措施。在研究可注射骨修复材料的固化性能时，相同组分和配方的材料有时候固化时间竟然不一样，多次重复实验，结果依然。这是一个令人头疼的问题，但也是一个十分有趣的现象。虽然令我百思不得其解，但激起了我的好奇心，一定要搞清楚什么原因使得这种现象产生。因为固化性能主要得益于半水硫酸钙，于是我用半水硫酸钙做重复实验，研究其固化性能。分析两次固化实验的异同之处发现，重复第二次实验时，使用的半水硫酸钙是相同的，进行实验的容器也是相同的，不同之处仅仅是进行第二次重复实验时使用了第一次实验的容器，但是容器没有洗刷掉第一次半水硫酸钙固化后的残余物。难道是这些残余物在起作用？带着这个问题，我又重复了实验，发现的确是这些残余物可以缩短半水硫酸钙的固化时间。这些残余物是半水硫酸钙水化后形成的二水硫酸钙，难道少量的二水硫酸钙可以促进半水硫酸钙的凝固？带着这个问题，我在半水硫酸钙中加入二水硫酸钙，继续进行固化实验，发现半水硫酸钙的固化性能确实得到改善，大大缩短了固化时间。基于这个发现，启发我在硫酸钙-矿化胶原可注射骨修复材料中加入二水硫酸钙作为促凝剂，果然使得材料的固化时间大大缩短。根据材料中二水硫酸钙和矿化胶原比例的不同，材料的固化时间可以根据需要在几分钟至100多分钟之间进行调节，大大提高了可注射骨修复材料的固化性能和应用性能，为以后的应用奠定了坚实的基础。这也许是在这个课题研究过程中一个最有意思的发现，依然得益于先生的醍醐灌顶。

3. 延续有前景的研究工作

在读博期间，我主要从事静电纺丝生物材料的研究工作。来到清华大学后，由于开始可注射骨修复材料的研究，博士期间从事的胶原-壳聚糖静电纺丝纳米纤维生物材料的相关研究暂告一段落。基于静电纺丝纳米纤维特殊的理化性能，静电纺丝纳米纤维作为生物材料也是一个有意义和前景的研究方向。先生了解我的这个研究领域，鼓励我继续把这个工作延续下去。基于先生的鼓励，我把问题进一步延伸，在此基础上提出了胶原-多糖仿生软组织细胞外基质的想法。对胶原-多糖仿生组织细胞外基质的理化性能进行了进一步研究和检测，以此进一步研究胶原-壳聚糖纳米纤维仿生细胞外基质对细胞生长的相关调控作用，发现了细胞在材料上有很好的黏附和生长行为，不同蛋白/多糖比例的材料对血管内皮细胞和平滑肌细胞有不同的调控行为。基于静电纺丝纳米纤维特殊的网络结构和高比表面积，细胞还可以进入纤维基质材料网络内部进行立体迁移生长，这对于细胞立体迁移、生长成为新的组织是重要的支持。这项工作依然得益于先生的支持和鼓励。

4. 回首昨天，展望明天

回顾在清华大学做博士后的日子，尤其是在先生的指导下，受益匪浅，对我来说是一笔无形的财富。先生的言传身教，不仅向我进一步诠释了踏实、勤恳、努力做人的道理，而且让我更深刻地理解了如何做一个科研人的真谛。同时，我也延续了当时在清华大学做博士后期间的一些科研工作。当然，这种延续是一种发展基础上的延续。我现在山东大学国家糖工程技术研究中心从事与糖相关的一些生物材料的研究工作。糖与核酸、蛋白质共同组成了生命体中最重要的3类生物大分子。研究发现，人类基因组表达产物中，至少一半是糖修饰产物。几乎所有的细胞表面和蛋白都含有糖链，加之细胞膜磷脂双分子层中含有大量的糖脂，使细胞表面覆盖了一层稠密的糖链，同时细胞赖以生长的微环境——细胞外基质也含有很多糖链。无疑，细胞表面及其周围大量糖链的存在，对于细胞与细胞及细胞与周围基质的相互作用是至关重要的。近年来，大量的研究表明，糖链及其缀合物在几乎所有的生理和病理过程中都发挥了极为重要的作用。与核酸和蛋白的生物合成不同，糖链的合成不是由固定的模板指导控制的，其表达具有时空特异性，即在不同的细胞和组织中，在不同的生理和病理条件下合成的糖链在组成和结构上是不同的。细胞中多种因素的协同作用决定了糖链的最终结构，这种时空特异性修饰，使有限的基因组产物具有更为丰富多样的结构特性，实现了在特定条件下对修饰产物功能的精细调节。因此，研究特定条件下糖链修饰生物材料调控细胞和组织修复的行为，对于开发具有更精微功能的生物材料十分重要。糖对生物材料的修饰，对于生物材料的发展来说，或许是点睛之笔。

以此为记，感谢崔福斋老师，祝老师 70 岁生日快乐。

# 培养期间代表性文章

Chen Z G, Wang P W, Wei B, Mo X M, Cui F Z. Electrospun collagen-chitosan nanofiber: A biomimetic extracellular matrix for endothelial cell and smooth muscle cell. *Acta Biomaterialia*, 2010, 6 (2): 372-382.

**Abstract** Electrospinning of collagen and chitosan blend solutions in a 1, 1, 1, 3, 3, 3-hexafluoroisopropanol/trifluoroacetic acid (v/v, 90/10) mixture was investigated for the fabrication of a biocompatible and biomimetic nanostructure scaffold in tissue engineering. The morphology of the electrospun collagen-chitosan nanofibers was observed by scanning electron microscopy (SEM) and stabilized by glutaraldehyde (GTA) vapor via crosslinking. Fourier transform infrared spectra analysis showed that the collagen-chitosan nanofibers do not change significantly, except for enhanced stability after crosslinking by GTA vapor. X-ray diffraction analysis implied that both collagen and chitosan molecular chains could not be crystallized in the course of electrospinning and crosslinking, and gave an amorphous structure in the nanofibers. The thermal behavior and mechanical properties of electrospun collagen-chitosan fibers were also studied by differential scanning calorimetry and tensile testing, respectively. To assay the biocompatibility of electrospun fibers, cellular behavior on the nanofibrous scaffolds was also investigated by SEM and methylthiazol tetrazolium testing. The results show that both endothelial cells and smooth muscle cells proliferate well on or within the nanofiber. The results indicate that a collagen-chitosan nanofiber matrix may be a better candidate for tissue engineering in biomedical applications such as scaffolds.

引用次数：**104**

# 3.22 尝试、挑战与自我的寻找

连小洁

太原理工大学力学学院，太原

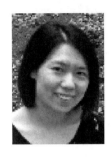

连小洁，2009 年 9 月—2012 年 8 月，在崔老师研究组从事博士后研究工作，博士后出站的论文题目是《抗感染骨修复材料的制备及性能研究》，出站后进入太原理工大学力学学院工作，副教授，硕士生导师。

　　从离开北京来到自己家乡的高校工作已经 3 年了，时间过得好快，这次有这样的机会把自己的学习经历以及受崔老师指导的经历写在崔老师的 70 岁生日纪念文集中是一件很荣幸的事情。边回顾边写，时间又回到了前几年在北京奋斗的日子。

　　我在北京理工大学获得博士学位，师从朱鹤孙先生（现在先生刚刚去世不久），进行的是 973 项目《丝素基材料的抗凝血材料改性及细胞在材料表面力学性能的研究》。博士毕业后要进行人生的一次重要选择，也有一些机会，可以选择继续做科研，进研究所或者读博士后。当时，我一直在思考一个问题：我做了 5 年的生物材料的基础研究，那么我做的材料除了动物实验，进一步更大的价值如何去实现，差距还有多大，距离还有多远。其实那个时候我很多做材料的同学，不只是生物材料，都有同样的困惑，我们的材料价值在哪里，基础研究和应用之间还需要多少年。现在回头来看，其实基础研究也是同样重要，但是当时的我，兴趣更多地集中在材料的产业化方面。当时，同学们纷纷地签约了。人才交流会我有时也会去，但是我更想从事生物材料相关的工作，但是发现并不是很多。无意中我看到招聘会中有一个公司，就是北京奥精医药科技有限公司，将生物材料产业化，而产品正是人工骨材料。当时第一感觉是终于找到了，而且觉得生物材料做成产品真是不容易，因为它是应用于人体的，需要更高的安全性。投简历后并没有及时反馈我，后来我从网上继续跟踪，然后打电话，公司终于约了我面试，没有想到的是，面试官竟然是清华大学材料科学与工程系的崔福斋教授。在面试中我第一次见到了崔老师、王秀梅老师（我博士后的合作导师）和胡堃博士。崔老师说："你可以读我们博士后的，博士来公司可惜了。"我当时说我想更多的从事产业化方面的工作。最后的结果是我读了清华的博士后，并且很大一部分时间在公司做一些工作。不得不说的是，崔老师给了我人生的一次很重要的机会。

在这 3 年中，崔老师帮我选了一个课题方向，就是抗感染骨修复材料。当时公司做的产品是崔老师其中的一个专利成果，集中了崔老师及研究组多少届师兄、师姐的辛苦和智慧，商品名叫做骼金，很好的名字，修复骨骼的"黄金"材料。我也参与了很多次该材料的研究，帮助公司做一些技术支持。这个材料的特点总体来说是仿生的结构（多孔）、仿生的成分（胶原和纳米羟基磷灰石），模拟了体内生物矿化过程，其强度接近松质骨，所以很有优势。我接触了很多骨科医生，崔老师给我提供了很多这样的机会，我也曾亲自去看材料植入的过程。很多代理商也和我沟通过，他们对这个材料采用的先进的科技及背后崔老师的专利技术感到很崇拜，很多人做这个产品的代理有很大一部分也是这个原因吧。在接触临床医生后我发现，他们很希望有针对治疗感染性骨缺损方面的材料，他们有具体的需求：构建一个局部药物释放系统（drug delivery system，DDS），通过载体将抗生素释入局部，可以在感染局部获得较高的血药浓度，且能够长期维持局部有效抑菌浓度，避免全身毒副反应，在抑制感染的同时实现对骨缺损的修复。他们谈到，只要药物能从载体释放 20 天就可以。而我们的材料的多孔结构，如果在制备过程中可以混入一些药物，或者在材料表面用浸渍法载药，都可以实现药物缓慢释放。同时，我们的材料本身具有优良的骨修复效果。基于这样的启发和思路，我们的第一部分研究工作开始了，这也是我博士后出站报告的第一部分内容——万古霉素复合胶原基骨修复材料的抗感染及骨修复性能研究。动物实验合作者是中国医科大学附属口腔医院的刘欢叶博士，实验的结果是除了保持原有胶原基骨修复材料（骼金）的多孔结构、高孔隙率及力学性能，材料的抑菌性能通过抑菌率试验和抑菌环试验进行检测，结果表明，材料对金黄色葡萄球菌作用 24 h，抑菌率大于 99%。材料在体外模拟体液中释放 30 天后药物浓度为 70 $\mu g/mL$，抑菌环直径为 （11.5±0.1） mm。材料能促进骨髓间充质干细胞的生长和黏附，植入材料 3 个月后，材料能抑制感染并且促进成骨。但由于时间关系，并没有进行长期的动物实验，基于载体材料的优良特性已经在很多研究和文献中得以证明，我对结果是乐观的。

还有一种材料是临床医生比较感兴趣的，同时，国外公司已有产品，就是以具有可注射性的半水硫酸钙为主要成分的材料。可塑型或者可注射是这一材料的最大优点，也是备受青睐的主要原因。我的博士后研究工作的另一内容便是万古霉素复合硫酸钙基骨修复材料的抗感染及骨修复性能研究，其中在半水硫酸钙凝固性能不受显著影响的基础上，我们用矿化胶原增加其生物活性，以此材料作为药物载体，构建药物缓释体系。在这一研究中，我的合作单位是中国人民解放军总医院毛克亚主任的研究组。动物实验仍然是3个月，从各种影像学和病理学检测结果来看，抗感染及骨修复效果还是比较好的。针对这一内容，我也以清华大学和北京奥精医药科技有限公司为发明人申请了一项发明专利。

博士后期间，我做得更多的是结合骨科临床的应用研究工作，也参与了奥精医药科技有限公司有关技术、销售等方面一些具体的工作，得到了很多的锻炼。在低头实验的过程中能够听一下医生的需求和建议，对我来说收获是比较大的。同时，进入清华大学崔老师的研究组，我体会比较深的就是崔老师的产业化魄力以及对外成功的交流与合作，开拓了我的视野，同时，对我日后的科研思路也产生了一定的影响。在这3年中，有很多的机会能和崔老师一起出去交流与合作，也深切地感受到崔老师严谨的科研态度以及不怕吃苦、孜孜以求的精神。

离开清华大学和崔老师，开始了自己新的独自的征程，在这个过程中仍然得到了崔老师、王老师以及同门师兄、师姐、师弟、师妹的帮助，以后的路唯有继续努力才不负清华精神及崔老师的指导。继续努力吧！

# 培养期间代表性文章

Lian X J, Liu H Y, Wang X M, Xu S J, Cui F Z, Bai X Z. Antibacterial and biocompatible properties of vancomycin-loaded nano-hydroxyapatite/collagen/poly (lactic acid) bone substitute. *Progress in Natural Science: Materials International*, 2013, 23 (6): 549-556.

**Abstract** Infected bone defects are normally regarded as contraindications for bone grafting. In the present study, an antibacterial bone graft substitute was synthesized by loading vancomycin (VCM) in our previously developed inineralized collagen based composite, nano-hydixixyapatite/collagen/poly (lactic acid) (nHAC/PLA), aiming to repair large size bone defects and inhibit related infections simultaneously. The VCM/nHAC/PLA showed typical porous structure with a porosity of (80.7 ± 6.7)% and compressive strength of 1.52 MPa. The delivery of VCM from VCM/nHAC/PLA was detected in vitro for up to 4 weeks, And their antibacterial properties were determined using inhibition ratio assay and inhibition zone assay. Pretty high level of inhibition ratio (more than 99%) was obtained in VCM/nHAC/PLA group. Additionally, a distinct inhibition zone was clearly formed in Staphylococcus aureus bacterium incubation dish with VCM/nHAC/PLA disc for up to 18 days of incubation. Moreover, both of the nHAC/PLA composites with or without VCM exhibited favorable in vitro and in vivo biocompatibilities for rabbit marrow stromal cells (MSCs) adhesion, spreading, proliferation, and triggering no obvious inflammation responses in subcutaneous implantation. Our results suggested that the VCM/nHAC/PEA performed ideal antibacterial property and biocoinpatibility and has great promise for the treatment of bone defect-related infections in orthopedic surgeries.

引用次数: 8

# 3.23　难忘师恩，难忘清华

## 于晓龙

海南大学材料与化工学院，海口

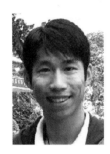

于晓龙，海南大学材料与化工学院教授，硕士生导师。2010年1月—2012年4月，在崔老师的研究组从事博士后研究工作，博士后出站的论文题目是《化学基团对肝癌细胞行为的影响》。

　　从清华大学出站至今已3年有余，然而，回想当年在清华大学材料科学与工程系学习的日子仍历历在目，崔老师的谆谆教诲仍时常回想在耳边，催我进取，教我踏实做事。

　　记得刚入站的时候，我草草收拾了行装奔赴清华大学，那是多少学子心目中梦寐的高校，尤其是可以师从生物材料领域的著名科学家崔福斋教授，心中无比兴奋，但同时也忐忑不安，不知自己能否完成学业，合格出站，也不知自己能否胜任这份工作。来到清华大学，初见了崔老师，他很关切地询问我吃饭和住宿安排的情况，我便一一作答，心中放下了包袱，原来崔老师如此和蔼可亲，平易近人，对我一个陌生且初来的学生如此关心。然而，我心中最大的忧虑是我的科研方向——生物材料学。毕竟我是学习凝聚态物理出身的学生，导师定给我的博士后课题是《化学基团对肝癌细胞行为的影响》，而我对该领域一无所知，直接和崔老师表示了我心中的疑虑。老师安慰我说：虽然我的基础专业距离生物材料有一定差距，但也属于该交叉学科需要的基础知识。如果说凝聚态物理是对无机世界的探索，对于我一个有博士研究能力的人而言，也可以同样做好生物材料领域的研究，世上无难事只要肯登攀。这一席话给了我莫大的鼓舞。然后崔老师带着我见了其他材料科学与工程系的合作导师，并不厌其烦地一一向对方介绍我的情况。填写了自己的入站申请书，自此我走入了生物材料研究的领域。

开始科研工作之初，由于我基础知识欠缺，实验能力不足，崔老师在百忙之中抽出时间带我进实验室手把手指导我的工作，还特意安排了几位师弟、师妹与我一同探索实验。即使我们的实验慢慢走上了轨道，他还是坚持调研一些我研究领域里面前沿的实验成果与我们讨论。在每周的讨论当中，我们都发现崔老师的科研敏感度极高，他总能抓住实验工作中最有科研价值的科学问题，点出其中的症结，并据此指导我们的实验方向。心中佩服之情油然而生，同时也鞭策自己要努力工作，莫辜负师恩。

入站后的日子里，崔老师的刻苦工作态度和科研精力更是令我由衷钦佩。在我负责 973 项目结题的财务工作时，经常遇到一些难于解决的事务，而且经常由于工作进度紧凑，需要在午休甚至深夜的时候向崔老师汇报情况，然而，老师每次都会很迅速地接听电话，并给我指导工作，其中有一次我们电话交流到凌晨 2 点。自此之后我对自己的工作进度再也不敢偷懒拖拉，时刻以老师的工作态度鞭策自己。还有一次，我与老师出差去希腊参加科研会议，旅途的颠簸与劳顿对于上了年纪的崔老师而言无疑是身体上的折磨。当时，我们在莫斯科机场转机的时候他已疲惫不堪，我就跟老师说："要不我们休息一天，改天再返程，"崔老师立即正色道："晚一天回去就耽误了一天的工作啊。"至今那难忘的旅程和简短的语言依然刻在我脑海里，催我进取，不敢懈怠。

两年的博士后工作中，最难忘的还是崔老师对学术问题的明智与坚持。我的研究工作中涉及自组装单分子膜的制备，这种单分子膜是用来充当我们研究肝癌细胞行为的载体，提供单一化学因素影响的微环境。我们已经在预实验中观测到了不同化学基团对相同的肝癌细胞是有不同影响的，我们都单纯地以为不同影响就单方面来自不同化学基团，而没有深究其他问题。崔老师询问道，会不会因为化学基团的面密度不同而带来不同影响呢？我们都无言以对，同时心里也惴惴不安，悔恨自己没有深入考虑。老师要求我们深入研究化学基团的面密度，我采用 X 射线光电子能谱法加以理论分析计算，近似阐述了不同化学基团的面密度基本相同。然而，崔老师批评我的科研态度不严谨，指出推测的理论计算不能根本性的说明该问题，必须使用显微镜。由于单分子膜工艺的限制，只能通过原子力显微镜来表征化学基团面密度，并且化学基团间距的理论值为 0.5 nm，这已经达到了原子力显微镜测试的极限，观测到清晰面密度图案的可能性极小，对实验难度和实验周期要求很高。我们尝试了多次都以失败告终，一度我都以为这个实验结果是做不出来的。但崔老师严谨的治学态度感染着我们，最后，他联系到华南理工大学杜昶教授帮助我。在杜教授的协助下，我们终于测到了理想的结果，当时的开心之情溢于言表。这是我人生第一次用坚持的态度完成了"不可能"的任务。

毕业出站，离开清华大学和崔老师，开始了自己新的征程，每年但凡有科研会议的机会，我都会赶去见见崔老师，体会那影响我终身的清华精神。愿崔老师永远身体健康，清华精神永存。

# 培养期间代表性文章

Yu X L, Zhang B, Wang X M, Wang Y, Qiao L, He J, Wang J, Chen S F, Lee I S, Cui F Z. Cancer cell proliferation controlled by surface chemistry in its microenvironment. *Frontiers of Materials science*, 2011, 5 (4): 412-416.

**Abstract**  Hepatoma cells (Hepg2s) as typical cancer cells cultured on hydroxyl (—OH) and methyl (—$CH_3$) group surfaces were shown to exhibit different proliferation and morphological changes. Hepg2s cells on —OH surfaces grew much more rapidly than those on —$CH_3$ surfaces. Hepg2s cells on —OH surfaces had the larger contact area and the more flattened morphology, while those on —$CH_3$ surfaces exhibited the smaller contact area and the more rounded morphology. After 7 days of culture, the migration of Hepg2s cells into clusters on the —$CH_3$ surfaces behaved significantly slower than that on the —OH surfaces. These chemically modified surfaces exhibited regulation of Hepg2s cells on proliferation, adhesion, and migration, providing a potential treatment of liver cancer.

# 3.24 上善若水，厚德载物

陶春生

中国人民解放军第 401 医院，青岛

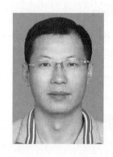 陶春生，1999 年，毕业于第二军医大学，分配到中国人民解放军第 401 医院工作；2002—2007 年，在第二军医大学附属长征医院骨科硕博连读；2012 年，进入清华大学材料学院，从事博士后研究，研究课题是《矿化胶原复合 PM-MA 骨水泥的改性研究》，2014 年出站。现为中国人民解放军第 401 医院骨科副主任医师，从事骨科临床工作。

今天看到崔福斋老师对孔子"温故而知新"这句名言的独到理解和诠释，很有感触，我想这应该是崔老师结合自己多年工作、学习过程中对科研精神和学习方法的切身感悟和总结。时值 70 岁生日之际，崔老师创造性地提出了"温故而知创新"的新语则更是对年轻科研人寄予了殷切的期望，这既是崔老师自己对科研创新精神的深刻体会，更是给年轻科研人指明了科学研究的方法和方向，可谓用心良苦。

实事求是地讲，我不算真正的科研人，但作为骨科医生，我深知科研创新对医学进步的重大影响，尤其是材料学的发展对骨科学的极大促进作用。回顾过去骨科学领域近 20 年里程碑式的改变，无论是治疗理念、手术水平还是治疗方法等方面都取得了前所未有的飞跃发展。诚然，这离不开骨科医生们的不懈努力和追求，但如果没有骨科相关材料学的革新，骨科整体医疗水平的提高便无从提起。在诸多的骨科材料学的革新中，清华大学崔福斋教授科研团队自主研发的矿化胶原基人工骨修复材料就是其中之一。这种人工骨材料是一种新型生物矿化的骨修复材料，与自体骨具有相同的成分和结构，不存在异体骨和异种骨的抗原性和交叉感染的问题，同时避免了取自体骨的痛苦和相关并发症，且临床治疗效果与自体骨可完全媲美，这为骨科临床骨缺损修复、脊柱融合等问题的解决带来了极大的便利。

我是 2012 年经过崔福斋老师的引领，有幸进入清华大学材料学院博士后流动站深造，在崔老师耳濡目染、言传身教的指导下，我对矿化胶原基骨生物材料进行了临床应用研究，并获得了一定的科研成果。此时，崔老师在生物材料学界的声名早已享誉中外，成就斐然，并取得了矿化胶原基人工骨修复材料等科研成果的成功产品转化并投放市场，这对于一个科研人来说，是非常不容易的，也是绝对了不起的。尽管获得了如此辉煌的成就和声誉，但在科研工作中，崔老师仍然保持着严谨科学、求真务实的科研人学风和作风，用"温故而知创新"的科研精神和学习方法影响着身边每一位年轻科研人的成长和进步，这让我也受益匪浅。与科研工作中的一丝不苟和严厉不同的是，在生活中，崔老师豁达开朗、温和、谦逊，乐于助人，我想这完全是崔老师善良的本性使然。这让每一位与之接触的人，都会感受到他自然而强大的亲和力和亲切感。时至今日，尽管崔老师早已功成名就、桃李满天下，而且昔日的很多弟子现在也已成为其相关研究领域的领军人物，但无论毕业早晚，离他远近，我们都仍然能够感受到崔老师对弟子们的关心、支持和殷切期望。

上善若水，厚德载物。这正是崔老师像水一样高尚的情操和像大地一样深厚的胸怀，滋养万物、包容万物、承载万物、造福万物而不求回报的真实写照。谨以此献给崔福斋老师 70 岁生日。

# 培养期间代表性文章

Tao C S, Qiu Z Y, Meng Q Y, Wu J J, Liu F, Wang C M, Cui F Z. Mineralized collagen incorporated polymethyl methacrylate bone cement for percutaneous vertebroplasty and percutaneous kyphoplasty. *Journal of Biomaterials and Tissue Engineering*, 2014, 4 (12): 1100-1106.

**Abstract** Polymethyl methacrylate (PMMA) is a bone cement materials commonly used by percutaneous vertebroplasty (PVP) and percutaneous kyphoplasty (PKP) in the treatment of vertebral body compression fracture. The safety, effectiveness and long-term curative effect of the PMMA bone cement have been verified with a lot of theoretical researches and clinical practices. However, in recent years, it has been reported that PMMA bone cement in vertebroplasty operation may cause some complications, such as adjacent vertebral fracture, and set PMMA bone cement may be loosened or even get off from the vertebral body. The high elastic modulus of PMMA would result in adjacent vertebral body fracture. On the other hand, bioinert PMMA cannot form osteointegration with autologous bone tissue, thereby the set PMMA bone cement is easy to be loosened or get off from the vertebral body. In this study, we used mineralized collagen (MC) with good osteogenic activity to develop a new composite PMMA vertebroplasty bone cement. As the content of MC reached

15 wt% in the powder part of the cement, the compressive modulus of the set bone cement was significantly reduced compared to pure PMMA bone cement and commercially available products, while the compressive strength maintained well. The MC incorporated PMMA bone cement also exhibited better cell compatibility and osteointegration ability.

# 3.25　三维结构组织工程支架的开发

## 孟庆圆

中国科学院遗传与发育生物学研究所，北京

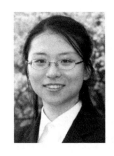

孟庆圆，2001—2005 年，就读于清华大学材料科学与工程系，获得学士学位；2005—2008 年，分别就读于清华大学材料科学与工程系和日本东京工业大学高分子科学系，同时获得两个硕士学位；2008—2012 年，就读于日本东京工业大学生体分子机能系，获得博士学位，从事细胞识别性基底材料诱导胚胎干细胞分化的研究。在 *Biomaterials*、*Journal of the American Chemical Society* 等国际期刊上发表文章 3 篇。2012—2015 年，在清华大学材料学院做博士后研究期间，从事水凝胶材料促进中枢神经修复和材料表面改性调控干细胞行为和功能方面的研究。2015 年至今，在中国科学院遗传与发育生物学研究所工作，从事 3D 生物打印方面的研究。

"温故而知创新"，源于孔子的"温故而知新"，其原意是熟悉已有的知识，在此基础上学会并掌握新知识。"温故而知创新"的含义是在熟悉、了解、掌握前人的研究基础上，创新发展，掌握新知识和新技术，开拓新理念和新领域，取得新进展和新成就。

我进入崔老师实验室的学习、研究以及工作经历，正体现了崔老师所倡导的"温故而知创新"这一理念。在本科进入实验室后，以及在硕士学习期间，包括随后的博士、博士后，乃至现在的研究工作阶段，我主要进行的研究内容就是对三维结构组织工程支架的开发。组织工程支架，顾名思义，就是由生物材料所构成的细胞支架，可与各种活细胞以及生物活性因子相结合，在植入生物体的缺损区域后提供一个人工的细胞外基质，吸引周围细胞的长入，诱导种子细胞增殖和分化，从而达到组织修复再生的目的。现有的组织工程支架已经被应用于骨、软骨、血管、神经、皮肤、肝、脾、肾及膀胱等组织器官。

我所做的研究就是根据生物体植入部位的特点，来设计三维支架的结构和功能，从而满足植入体内的需要，其内容涉及血管、尿道、神经、肝脏等多个组织器官。在此就以小血管为例，分享一下我的研究经历。血管即血液流过的管道，几乎遍布人体各处，一旦发生狭窄或阻塞，可能会造成很严重的后果。现有的人工血管开发多是基于尼龙、涤纶及聚四氟乙烯等人工合成材料。其中，大、中口径的人工血管已经在临床上取得了较为满意的效果，但是小血管的研发仍然存在着比较大的问题。当时从崔老师手里接到这个研究课题，也是一头雾水，对这个领域已用的研究成果和发展方向没有一点了解。崔老师要求我要通读这一领域的相关文献，了解已有研究的进展，对前人工作的优、缺点要做到心中有数。果然，在阅读了大量的资料以后，我对小血管支架的研究有了足够的认识，最终选择了电纺丝方法制备聚乳酸血管支架。当时的研究条件还比不上现在，国内还没有成熟的电纺丝设备，国外的仪器价格昂贵，到货周期长得让人绝望。于是，在又一轮调研后，我们选择了自己搭建设备。一个高压电源、一套针头改装的注射装置、手工打造的接收板组合起来就是我们的电纺丝机器。为了确保实验安全，我们把机器安置在一个通风橱里，占据了实验室的一个角落；高压地线接在暖气的金属板上，然后立起一块"注意安全"的牌子，这就是我们实验的场地。我们研究了电压、溶液浓度、接收距离等多种条件对电纺性能的影响。为了观察电纺丝的实时效果，要把脑袋凑到设备前面观察。有时候，电纺出的纤维丝喷得满头满脸都是，而我们却会为了测试出一个满意的参数而兴高采烈。可是，为了得到一个能耐受体内压力的管状结构，手工打制的小接收板就不能满足要求了。于是，我们再次投身文献的海洋，在前人的工作里寻找灵感，最后，搭建出一个小型的旋转接收装置，可以无缝接收材料，得到我们需要的结构。随后的测试过程也体现出"温故而知创新"的理念。我们通过调研，设计出自己的水压测试系统，模拟出类似体内的环境，从而测试出三维血管支架对血压的耐受能力。这种"温故而知创新"的精神鼓励我在今后的科研工作中不断追求。随后在日本读研究生阶段，我所进行的利用基底材料诱导调控干细胞生长和定向分化的工作，取得了很好的结果，发表在 *Biomaterials*、*Journal of the American Chemical Society* 等期刊上，也取得了日本《读卖新闻》等大众媒体的关注。

在研究工作中，我们在不断地开发新的组织工程产品，希望能够造福人类，提高人类的生活质量。我们在研究中，不断地遇到新的难题，又在前人的激励中解决问题。我们是"站在巨人肩膀上"的一代人，前人的基础和成果给我们指明了后面研究的方向。从李恒德先生到崔老师，再到我们，科研精神的火炬就这么一代代地传下去。在这短暂的研究生涯中，我不断地在研究探索中找到乐趣；在日常工作中，找到妙趣；在攻关克服困难中，找到兴趣，支持我走下去。

# 培养期间代表性文章

Meng Q Y, Tao C S, Qiu Z Y, Akaike T, Cui F Z, Wang X M. A hybrid substratum for primary hepatocyte culture that enhances hepatic functionality with low serum dependency. *International Journal of Nanomedicine*, 2015, 10: 2313-2323.

**Abstract**    Cell culture systems have proven to be crucial for the in vitro maintenance of primary hepatocytes and the preservation of hepatic functional expression at a high level. A poly-( N-p-vinylbenzyl-4-O-β-D-galactopyranosyl-D-gluconamide ) matrix can recognize cells and promote liver function in a spheroid structure because of a specific galactose-asialoglycoprotein receptor interaction. Meanwhile, a fusion protein, E-cadherin-Fc, when incubated with various cells, has shown an enhancing effect on cellular viability and metabolism. Therefore, a hybrid substratum was developed for biomedical applications by using both of these materials to combine their advantages for primary hepatocyte cultures. The isolated cells showed a monolayer aggregate morphology on the coimmobilized surface and displayed higher functional expression than cells on traditional matrices. Furthermore, the hybrid system, in which the highest levels of cell adhesion and hepatocellular metabolism were achieved with the addition of 1% fetal bovine serum, showed a lower serum dependency than the collagen/gelatin-coated surface. Accordingly, this substrate may attenuate the negative effects of serum and further contribute to establishing a defined culture system for primary hepatocytes.

# 3.26 让科学成果走出实验室

仇志烨

北京奥精医药科技有限公司

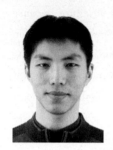

仇志烨，清华大学材料学院博士后。从事可降解仿生骨修复材料的研究和产品研发，与企业开展深度合作，主持研发和改进的部分产品已应用于临床，并获得良好评价；参与临床需求分析和产品推广等市场工作。申请并获批国家自然科学基金青年基金 1 项，中国博士后科学基金 1 项。入选北京市优秀人才。发表学术文章 10 余篇，申请国家发明专利多项。

从小到大，时常感慨于大自然的神奇——造就了生物体奇特的物质组成和美轮美奂的构造，以及令人匪夷所思的运行方式。我不禁思索，以人类文明的发展程度和速度，何时才能参透自然造化的神奇，又如何才能模仿甚至改进我们自身？随着学习的知识越来越多，这些疑问就愈发强烈。带着这样的好奇和憧憬，我选择了生物材料这门复杂且综合性极强的学科作为自己的研究生专业。学业成长中我越来越深刻地感觉到，大自然造就的人体真的是精妙绝伦，从物质到结构，从微观到宏观，复杂而又有序，每个器官、每块组织各司其职而又协同配合。于是，做研究的同时便也不断思考，若是能制造出与天然人体组织一模一样的仿生材料，哪怕是简单的单一组织，那将是多么完美的作品！而若是能将这些成果变成产品应用到临床，更会是一件富有挑战而意义非凡的事情。于是，整个研究生期间我参与了不少应用型的课题，研究了元素掺杂羟基磷灰石、多孔胶原支架、聚乳酸载药微球、壳聚糖神经导管等，以及一些生物材料的产业化工作。

初识崔老师是在 2007 年的中韩生物材料大会上。因为是我的博士导师张胜民教授主办此次会议，主场优势让我有幸聆听了包括崔老师在内的诸多领域专家的精彩报告，了解到许多学科发展和产业化的前沿，尤其对崔老师的仿生骨修复材料研究和产业化工作印象颇深。于是，在日后的学习中和学术会议等场合也对清华大学研究组的工作进展特别关注。机缘巧合，在接下来几年的

863 项目、"十二五"国家科技支撑计划等国家科研项目中，我都有幸代表张教授的研究组，与清华大学研究组的老师共同设计课题，并合作完成项目研究工作，期间也认识了研究组的不少老师，如冯庆玲教授、王秀梅老师等。

既然如此投缘，在获得博士学位后，带着崇敬、向往、好奇等复杂的情绪，我投身到崔老师门下，成为清华大学再生医学与仿生材料研究所的一员，开启了博士后的角色。记得初次与崔老师见面，被问及想做些什么，我直言想做生物材料的产品研发，出人意料地，崔老师爽快答应了，并安排我到合作企业——北京奥精医药科技有限公司开展工作，而这一安排，最终决定了我延续到今天的职业生涯，这是后话。满足个人发展愿望，宽松且人性化的环境，给了我广博的天地从事生物材料的科学研究和产品开发。平心而论，清华大学生物材料研究组实验室的硬件条件确实普通，实验室面积不大，仪器设备也有限，老师和学生却不少。然而，人的因素决定了一个团队的实力和层次。在这里，每一位老师都实力非凡，并且工作认真细致、孜孜不倦，高素质的学生也不断涌现。借助于清华大学优质的平台资源，崔老师的团队扬起了中国生物材料界的一面大旗，而这一切，无疑都源自于崔老师高深的学术造诣、对工作的严格要求和对团队的科学管理。

博士后工作期间，我深度参与到奥精医药科技有限公司的医疗器械产品的开发工作，也因此更多地接触了崔老师在医疗器械产品产业化方面的理念和思路。在生物材料产品的产业化实施过程中，崔老师制定的目标简单而明确，就是要把实验室产出的优质成果应用到临床，造福广大患者，解决临床实际需求。而同时，问题的解决方法，或者说产品开发和临床转化的具体操作方式和实现途径则是多种多样的。于是，在明确的目标导引下，辅之以灵活多样的方法和手段，汇集了崔老师 10 余年研究心血的明星材料——矿化胶原——成功实现了产业化。到如今已成功获得 3 项 CFDA 三类医疗器械产品注册证和 1 项美国 FDA 注册证，发展出的产品多达 30 余种，涵盖骨科、神经外科、口腔科、整形外科等诸多领域，临床使用 10 余万例，骨缺损修复效果良好。除了研发，我还与奥精医药科技有限公司市场部、销售部紧密配合，参与了产品的医院科室宣讲会、学术推广等方面的工作，积累了不少市场经验。并与许多医生深入交流临床遇到的问题，分析需求，制定产品研发和改进方案。这些工作使我对医疗器械产品的需求分析和设计的关键环节有所了解和参与，受益匪浅。而这些经验的取得，也必须感谢崔老师的指引和信任。

崔老师非常注重对年轻人的培养，但凡领域内有价值的学术会议，崔老师都不吝啬机会，让学生们去更广阔的知识天地驰骋。崔老师还非常乐意利用自己的好人缘和学术地位，为学生们与领域内知名专家学者之间牵线搭桥，为年轻人提供更丰富的机会和道路选择。短短几年间，我也有幸陪同崔老师行便祖国大江南北，认识了许许多多科学家、医生、学者及政府人士等，也获得了不少展现自己的机会，不断促进工作的开展和自身水平的提高。崔老师不仅在专业上给学生以指导，其大家风范更向学生们言传身教了许多行事做人的道理和为人处世的法则，让我们受益终身。

值此崔老师 70 大寿之际，祝福崔老师身体健康，万事如意，福如东海，寿比南山！希望崔老师继续指引团队攀登新的高峰，在生物材料的科学研究和产业化发展道路上更进一步，再铸新的辉煌！

## 培养期间代表性文章

Qiu Z Y, Tao C S, Cui H, Wang C M, Cui F Z. High-strength mineralized collagen artificial bone. *Frontiers of Materials Science*, 2014, 8（1）: 53-62.

**Abstract**　Mineralized collagen（MC）is a biomimetic material that mimics natural bone matrix in terms of both chemical composition and microstructure. The biomimetic MC possesses good biocompatibility and osteogenic activity, and is capable of guiding bone regeneration as being used for bone defect repair. However, mechanical strength of existing MC artificial bone is too low to provide effective support at human load-bearing sites, so it can only be used for the repair at non-load-bearing sites, such as bone defect filling, bone graft augmentation, and so on. In the present study, a high strength MC artificial bone material was developed by using collagen as the template for the biomimetic mineralization of the calcium phosphate, and then followed by a cold compression molding process with a certain pressure. The appearance and density of the dense MC were similar to those of natural cortical bone, and the phase composition was in conformity with that of animal's cortical bone demonstrated by XRD. Mechanical properties were tested and results showed that the compressive strength was comparable to human cortical bone, while the compressive modulus was as low as human cancellous bone. Such high strength was able to provide effective mechanical support for bone defect repair at human load-bearing sites, and the low compressive modulus can help avoid stress shielding in the application of bone regeneration. Both in vitro cell experiments and in vivo implantation assay demonstrated good biocompatibility of the material, and in vivo stability evaluation indicated that this high-strength MC artificial bone could provide long-term effective mechanical support at human load-bearing sites.

# 3.27 我在清华生物材料组的那三年

## 陈 曦

墨尔本大学，澳大利亚

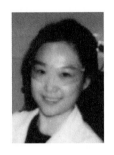

陈曦，2005—2009 年，就读于吉林大学材料科学与工程学院，主修无机非金属材料工程。大学四年成绩全系第一，多次获得校奖学金，2008 年获国家奖学金。2008 年，免试保送到清华大学材料科学与工程系。2009—2012 年，就读于清华大学材料科学与工程系生物材料研究组。2011 年 6 月，前往加拿大阿尔伯塔大学进行短期交换学习。2012—2016 年，就读于澳大利亚墨尔本大学化学与生物分子工程系，从事纳米材料癌症治疗方向的学习和研究。

很高兴收到崔福斋老师和王秀梅老师的邀请，简短回顾我在清华大学生物材料组学习和科研的时光。

2009 年 2 月，还在大四本科阶段的我，提前进入了生物材料组进行本科毕业课题的设计与研究。记得那时候整个组，包活崔老师、王老师、孙老师及蔡老师的所有学生一起召开大组会，每个学生轮流报告自己近期的实验进展。当时，由于本科专业是无机非金属材料的合成，我对于材料在生物体内的应用很是陌生。

2009 年 9 年，作为一名研究生新生，我开始了硕士阶段的学习。第一学年，为了弥补自己在生物材料学方面的不足，我选修了几乎所有能选修的生物材料相关的课程，包括生物材料、组织工程、生化实验及药物递送等。短短一学期的课程，使我基本上了解了生物材料学方面的知识架构。

这其中，印象最深刻的一门课就是崔老师的生物材料学。之所以对其印象深刻，是因为这门课的期末考试是基于对一种生物材料产品的设计报告。当时，还是新生的我，与核材料组的黄亮、陈诗蕾 3 个人走进了崔老师的办公室。那应该是我第一次进崔老师的办公室，满墙都是师兄、师姐博士答辩时和崔老师的合影，当时就想我何时能博士毕业。崔老师布置给我们的课题是可降解的镁合金血管支架。拿到课题后，我们 3 个人分工布置分课题的调研。陈诗蕾负责镁及其合金材料的调研，黄亮负责支架的工程制图，我负责可降解血管支架材料的调研。经过快 3 周的收集材料和反复讨论，我们设计出两种材料设计方案，并提交了课程报告——《两种用于小血管修复的新型镁合金固定支架材料设计方案》。最终，我拿到了整个课程的最高分数 91 分，同时相应的设计产品也投入到了下一步的研究。通过这门课，使我对生物体有了深入的了解和认识，也发挥了自己在材料设计上的优势。也许就是从那个时候起，我开始喜欢上了生物材料这个多领域交叉的学科。

2010 年 9 月起，我开始了硕士课题的研究工作，我拟做的硕士课题是《介孔二氧化硅的形貌控制及其在和细胞相互作用时的影响》。但是由于当时介孔二氧化硅的生物应用还未在组内开展，我很遗憾没有深入研究相关的生物学实验，因此最终的硕士论文题目是《共缩聚法制备形貌可控的介孔二氧化硅纳米材料》。虽然没有亲自完成介孔材料生物应用的工作，但近年来大量相关工作在国际高水平的学术期刊报道，也验证了当初选题的正确性。

感谢崔老师在硕士学习阶段对我的帮助，先后建议和推荐我去加拿大及荷兰进行学习。2011 年 6 月—9 月，作为国际短期交换生，我前往加拿大阿尔伯塔大学学习。第一次走出国门去发达国家，我见识到了与国内不同的学习氛围和校园文化，坚定了我出国攻读博士学位的想法。2012 年硕士毕业后，由于对生物材料这个学科的喜欢，我加入墨尔本大学化学与生物分子工程系，从师于澳洲科学院院士 Prof. Frank Caruso，从事纳米材料癌症治疗方向的研究至今。

回想在清华生活、学习和科研的时光，感恩崔老师把我从一个懵懂本科生带入了生物材料这个充满魅力和挑战的学科。感谢蔡老师、王老师和孙老师对我们学生的指导。我十分庆幸自己可以和一群充满朝气的同伴一起学习和交流。清华三年，我大大提高了自己在科研方向的整体把握和实验方案设计的能力，这也是我能够完成博士学习的很重要的原因之一。

对于科研创新，我认为没有对课题整个相关科研背景的全面了解和认识，是很难在他人工作基础上开展创新性工作的。所以在开展课题前，进行系统性地深入调研，是必不可少的。在别人工作的基础之上，找到可以突破或创新的地方，进而明确自己工作的意义，设计实验方案，积极与同学或导师讨论实验方案的可行性。最后，系统化定性和定量地开展实验。好的科研成果应该是对其他人的工作有指导性的，同时，能够让他人重复出自己的实验是至关重要的。实验的创新性源于自己对实验的细微观察和思考，因为只有自己的观察才是最与众不同的。

生物材料这个学科是多学科交叉的领域，涉及材料学、生物学、医学、化学和物理学等学科，我们都在努力地学习各方面的知识，完善每一个科研细节，这其中需要与来自不同学科背景的人深入交流和合作，大家毫无保留地交换想法和意见，将会使整个学科向实际临床应用更近一步。

最后，再次感谢恩师崔老师对我的帮助和指导，在老师 70 岁生日之际，祝您身体健康，吉祥喜乐，桃李天下。

# 3.28 化学功能团调控碳酸钙结晶成核的仿生矿化研究历程

## 邓 华

### 杰克逊州立大学，美国

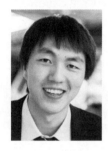

邓华，2009 年，本科毕业于中央民族大学生命与环境科学学院化学专业；2009—2012 年，广西师范大学与清华大学联合培养硕士研究生；2010—2013 年，在清华大学崔福斋教授、广西师范大学沈星灿教授共同指导下开展碳酸钙仿生矿化研究，完成毕业论文《化学功能团调控碳酸钙结晶受钙离子浓度影响的机理研究》。2013 年至今，在杰克逊州立大学攻读博士学位，从事抗耐药细菌纳米材料的开发和改性的相关研究。

崔福斋教授的生物材料研究组一直以来在生物矿化方面有很深的研究，尤其是通过胶原调控磷酸钙的仿生矿化研究，首次在纳米级别观察到类似骨晶体学取向的结构，对于骨修复和再生有重要意义。对所有的高等动物而言，骨和牙最主要的化学成分都是磷酸钙（羟基磷灰石），而骨、牙形成最开始的原料来源是磷酸根离子和钙离子。钙离子、磷酸根离子及胶原等在人体生理环境下，通过各种"生物因子"的调控作用，从磷酸钙的晶格取向开始形成纳米级的骨单元，并从微米到毫米甚至米尺度上进行严格地顺序组装和排列，最终生长成为特定形状、硬度和功能的肉眼能分辨的骨结构。

在临床研究方面，骨和牙的原位诱导再生一直是世界性难题。而解开这个难题的钥匙在于弄清钙离子等各种原材料从离子到纳米到微米，最终到宏观材料，一级一级组装形成的详细机理和过程。然而，关于钙离子、磷酸根离子等生物矿化形成骨、牙的很多细节过程仍然是个谜。实际上，全球很多科学家致力于研究骨、牙形成，但由于生物体环境中涉及太多复杂因素的参与，包括各种体液中存在分子级别的化学物质、生物体细胞甚至组织，直接人体模拟磷酸钙矿化几乎是不可能实现的。此外，由于磷酸钙有多种晶型，例如三磷酸钙、磷酸八钙、透磷石、单斜磷酸钙等，在离子形成结晶的过程中，想要完美调控磷酸钙形成成骨所需要的羟基磷灰石更是十分困难。

在这种情况下，我们把注意力转向了磷酸钙的"近亲"——碳酸钙。碳酸钙在自然界中存在更为广泛，是各种岩石和天然矿石的主要成分，更重要的是，碳酸钙是组成低等动物体内钙化产物的主要成分，例如海洋动物骨骼、耳石以及珍珠等。这些生物体内的碳酸钙通常都是特定单晶碳酸钙（方解石）或者具有特定排列的晶体结构，这些结构组成不同位置通常都有特定的功能，包括支撑、重力感应和传感、光学作用等，对动物体生命的维持和对环境的适应都起着举足轻重的作用。与磷酸钙一样，碳酸钙的生物矿化的很多细节也是未解之谜。而且，高等动物体内磷酸钙的生物矿化和低等动物体内碳酸钙的生物矿化必然有很多联系和相似之处。因此，体外仿生模拟碳酸钙的生物矿化必然会带给磷酸钙生物矿化机理全新的认识。

相对于磷酸钙而言，碳酸钙的同素异构体较少，最常见的生物矿物沉淀析出的有3种晶相：方解石、文石和球文石。热力学稳定性从强至弱依次为方解石、文石和球文石。鉴于碳酸钙在自然界中广泛存在而且具有确定的结构形式，碳酸钙结晶一直是生物矿化领域一个重要的研究方向，也是我们选择碳酸钙作为研究动物体内钙盐生物矿化例子的主要原因。

选择碳酸钙作为研究生物矿化的目标之后，下一个问题是如何实现所谓的"仿生"，即尽可能地模拟生物体内环境调控碳酸钙的结晶过程。如同以上所述的生物生命体系的复杂性，直接模拟体液环境是不可能实现的。在实验室条件下的能模仿的因素也是十分单一。同时，崔福斋教授提出，从原材料入手，最开始与离子相互作用的必然是分子水平上的结构。任何生物体系内的调控因子，无论是化学分子还是细胞乃至组织，与离子相互作用直接关联的必然是化学功能团。考虑到生物体内矿化可能涉及的调控因子——氨基酸或蛋白质，因此，我们选择了最常见的 4 种末端功能团：羧基（—COOH）、氨基（—$NH_3$）、羟基（—OH）和甲基（—$CH_3$），从分子水平模拟碳酸钙的结晶成核过程。

在研究方法方面，由于单个功能团对钙离子的作用很微小，无法观察和记录。为了解决这个问题，我们采用化学功能团的自组织单分子层膜，将化学功能团的作用放大，然后从纳米和微米尺度来观察碳酸钙结晶的区别，进而从分子水平认识各种功能团从最初期对钙盐生物矿化的调控。结果表明，这是个可行有效的仿生模拟方法。

在一年多的研究过程中，尽管我们遇到了很多方法上的和检测手段上的局限，但通过对实验各个细节上的不断改进，我们观察到了化学功能团和钙离子浓度共同调控碳酸钙初期结晶成核的不同现象。该部分成果发表在英国皇家化学会的 *Cryst. Eng. Comm.* 上。

该文章系统报道了不同功能团调控碳酸钙结晶的不同现象和结果，同时指出了钙离子浓度在其中也有重要的作用。之前也有各种关于功能团调控碳酸钙结晶的报道，但是不同报道之间结果差异很大甚至矛盾，该文章则比较系统地分析比较了各种功能团调控的结果。

然而，观察到调控结果和我们的研究碳酸钙生物矿化机理细节的方向还相差很远。我们在之前的实验基础上，进一步选择和优化实验条件，并引入钙离子电极来监测整个碳酸钙结晶过程中钙离子浓度的变化。最终观察到两个核心细节：一是碳酸钙先形成小尺寸的无定形碳酸钙微粒，这些微粒在功能团表面聚集长大形成碳酸钙晶体；二是功能团极性及旋转控制碳酸钙从无定形转化成为晶体的取向和生长方向。该部分成果发表在牛津大学出版社的 *Regenerative Biomaterials* 上。

由于经典的矿化理论认为，晶体成核初期是由离子不断的添加和组合，其过程类似于"砖头砌墙"，而新兴的理论认为，是先在溶液中形成很小的粒子，粒子团聚，长大并结晶形成晶体。该文章证明了在各个功能团表面的最初期成核机理，指出在羧基表面有一部分晶体成核是通过经典理论实现的，但在其他功能团表面以及自然界体系各种功能团共同存在的条件下，成核结晶是通过粒子实现的。在这项研究期间，我们应邀为 Springer 出版社的 *Frontiers of Materials Science* 撰写了化学功能团调控碳酸钙结晶的综述。

我们完成了预想的研究，观察到了不同功能团对碳酸钙结晶的调控以及初期成核结晶的机理细节。但这整个研究的完成对于整个生物矿化领域来说，只是冰山一角。很多研究者一直在尝试设计不同的分子结构或者表面来调控碳酸钙（碳酸钙晶体相对容易控制）结晶形成特定的取向、形貌和尺寸。"控制"晶体生长的研究还会进行，不同的是设计者将逐渐从小分子或者表面的二维调控转向通过高分子（如蛋白质、高聚物等）实现三维的调控，三维体系将涉及更多的更复杂的调控因素，包括高分子的折叠结构、空间局限等，但三维体系也能更好地实现对晶体结构的人为的可控的调控。如果将三维体系放置于仿生体液或其他人为设计的液体甚至胶体环境中，这种模仿体系也更接近生物体内复杂的生物矿化环境。

此外，对碳酸钙、磷酸钙生物矿化的研究最直接的受益者是骨、牙的再生修复。这也是理论研究的一个最重要的目的之一。目前，已经有很多基于羟基磷灰石的诱导骨再生的商业产品，这些产品得益于不断的生物矿化研究，一直在经历着改进和完善，包括在操作性，生物相容性以及诱导骨再生效果等方面。但是，对牙相关产品的应用十分有限，都停留在牙的"周边产品"，因为目前为止还没法实现（成人）牙的再生。对牙相关产品的开发以及对牙再生的探索也是生物矿化研究的一个重要方向之一。

在过去几年的科研工作中，深深体会到研究和探索才能找到知识的源头。

对于研究生，好的导师和研究团队是迈入科研大门的推动者和保障。而作为科研工作者，对的方向和好的研究方案是成功的关键，这些来源于自己对该领域不断的认识和积累，以及与同行的广泛交流。细节往往是决定成败的关键之一，不断发现问题，改进细节和解决问题，是引导科研工作者走向正确结论的必经之路。同时，专心、专注研究，必然会有所收获。

# 培养期间代表性文章

1. Deng H, Wang X M, Du C, Shen X C, Cui F Z. Combined effect of ion concentration and functional groups on surface chemistry modulated CaCO$_3$ crystallization. *Cryst. Eng. Comm.*, 2012, 14 (20): 6647-6653.

**Abstract** The effects of self-assembled monolayer templates terminated with carboxyl, hydroxyl, amino and methyl groups (—COOH, —OH, —NH$_2$ and —CH$_3$) on CaCO$_3$ crystallization are compared in aqueous solutions of low, medium and high Ca$^{2+}$ concentrations. On the —COOH surface, only calcite rhombohedra are crystallized in the solutions at three different concentrations, while size, shape and orientation of the formed calcites are distinct in various Ca$^{2+}$ concentration solutions. In low Ca$^{2+}$ concentration solution, vaterites (111) and (200) are formed on —OH and —NH$_2$ surfaces respectively while no crystals are observed on —CH$_3$ surface. In high Ca$^{2+}$ concentration solution, calcite (104) is formed on the —OH surface. Calcites and small amounts of vaterites and aragonites are formed on —NH$_2$ and —CH$_3$ surfaces. In medium concentration solutions, the results are similar to the case of high concentration with a lower density of crystals. From the view of the two well-known mechanisms for biomineralization, ion absorption and particle-based crystallization, the results in our study are discussed. Our findings can advance the understanding of CaCO$_3$ biomineralization in nature and also supply guidance for the design of advanced biomaterials.

2. Deng H, Shen X C, Wang X M, Du C. Calcium carbonate crystallization controlled by functional groups: A mini-review. *Frontiers of Materials Science*, 2013, 7 (1): 62-68.

**Abstract** Various functional groups have been suggested to play essential roles on biomineralization of calcium carbonate (CaCO$_3$) in natural system. 2D and 3D models of regularly arranged functional groups have been established to investigate their effect on CaCO$_3$ crystallization. This mini-review summarizes the recent progress and the future development is prospected.

引用次数：**6**

3. Deng H, Wang S, Wang X M, Du C, Shen X C, Wang Y J, Cui F Z. Two competitive nucleation mechanisms of calcium carbonate biomineralization in response to surface functionality in low calcium ion concentration solution. *Regenerative Biomaterials*, 2015, 2 (3): 187~195.

**Abstract**  Four self-assembled monolayer surfaces terminated with —COOH, —OH, —NH$_2$ and —CH$_3$ functional groups are used to direct the biomineralization processes of calcium carbonate (CaCO$_3$) in low Ca$^{2+}$ concentration, and the mechanism of nucleation and initial crystallization within 12 h was further explored. On —COOH surface, nucleation occurs mainly via ion aggregation mechanism while prenucleation ions clusters may be also involved. On —OH and —NH$_2$ surfaces, however, nucleation forms via calcium carbonate clusters, which aggregate in solution and then are adsorbed onto surfaces following with nucleation of amorphous calcium carbonate (ACC). Furthermore, strongly negative-charged —COOH surface facilitates the direct formation of calcites, and the —OH and —NH$_2$ surfaces determine the formation of vaterites with preferred crystalline orientations. Neither ACC nor crystalline CaCO$_3$ is observed on —CH$_3$ surface. Our findings present a valuable model to understand the CaCO$_3$ biomineralization pathway in natural system where functional groups composition plays a determining role during calcium carbonate crystallization.

# 3.29 仿生法制备人工角膜支架生物活性涂层

## 王乐耘

上海交通大学材料科学与工程学院，上海

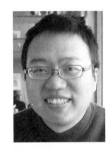

王乐耘，2003—2007 年，本科就读于清华大学材料科学与工程系，在崔福斋教授的指导下完成了本科毕业设计，参与了清华大学与中国人民解放军总医院的一项合作开发人工角膜的课题，负责角膜钛支架上的生物活性羟基磷灰石涂层设计，毕业论文题目为《仿生法制备羟基磷灰石涂层用于人工角膜支架》；2007—2011 年，在美国密歇根州立大学攻读博士学位，研究方向为金属钛晶粒尺度变形机理，2011 年被评为系优秀博士生。2011—2015 年，先后在美国阿贡国家实验室以及德国亥姆霍兹材料与海洋研究中心工作，研究领域包括同步辐射材料表征、核电用钢铁材料、稀土强化镁合金等方向。迄今为止在 *Acta Materialia*、*Scripta Materialia* 等国际期刊发表文章 15 篇，被引用 200 余次。2015 年，获得美国材料协会颁发的具有近百年历史的 Henry Marion Howe 最佳论文奖。2015 年底，作为特别研究员加入上海交通大学材料科学与工程学院。

    崔福斋教授是我在清华大学材料科学与工程系本科毕业设计的指导老师。这次能作为他的学生参与本纪念文集的撰写，我感到非常荣幸。尽管在崔老师研究组里仅工作了一年，但崔老师那时候的言传身教对我后来的成长有着巨大的影响。本文将主要回顾那一年我在崔老师的指导下完成的一个为人工角膜制备羟基磷灰石涂层的项目，那段经历让我至今难以忘怀。

    2006 年的夏天，当时大三的我们要选择生产实习的指导老师。生产实习本身是一门 5 学分的课，本科生通过加入一位老师的研究组来体验科研活动。当时我从未在课堂里接触过生物材料，对这个领域感到很新鲜，所以就给崔老师发了一封邮件，希望能加入他的研究组。崔老师收到邮件后，把我叫到他办公室聊了一会，然后就同意我加入了。

    暑假开始后，我到生物材料组里报道。一开始，崔老师让我跟着他的一位博士研究生做一个关于牙齿的课题。大概两周之后，我向崔老师邮件汇报了自己的学习进展，然后崔老师把我叫到他办公室，告诉我正好有一个和中国人民解放军总医院的关于人工角膜的合作项目，问我是否愿意参加。我欣然接受了这个能让我独立做点研究的项目，它后来也成为我生产实习以及本科毕业设计的主课题。

中国人民解放军总医院眼科在全国享有盛名，当时他们在黄一飞主任的领导下正在研发一款人工角膜。该角膜由光学元件以及支架两部分组成。其中光学元件是一块聚甲基丙烯酸甲酯柱状体，准备镶嵌在一片钛支架上植入人眼内。为了使整个装置能在眼球内固定，该设计要求在植入一段时间后，钛支架能与周围组织建立有机联系。为此，中国人民解放军总医院眼科委托清华大学生物材料组在他们提供的钛支架上沉积一层具有生物相容性的羟基磷灰石涂层，以诱导周围眼部组织将来在其表面生长。

崔老师把这项任务交给了我，并给我一篇他组里的硕士毕业论文作为学习文献。该论文主要讨论如何利用仿生法制备羟基磷灰石涂层。相比于离子束沉积法、电化学沉积法等工业常用涂层制备手段，仿生法模拟了自然界中天然生物材料的矿化、生长过程，对于制备羟基磷灰石涂层有一些独到的优越性，主要表现为：① 工艺简便，可在常温下进行；② 能够在形状复杂的试样表面制备均匀的涂层；③ 可进行微结构控制；④ 在涂层中引入生物活性分子更为方便。根据生物矿化原理，涂层仿生合成的思想是：使基体表面挂上功能性基团（预处理），然后浸渍入过饱和溶液，无机物在功能化表面以分子识别机理发生异相成核和生长，从而形成涂层。

我仔细研读了那篇硕士论文，根据里面提供的参数制定了一个涂层沉积的工艺：砂纸打磨→丙酮、乙醇、去离子水依次清洗→在 0.6 mol/L 的 NaOH 溶液中于 160 ℃下处理 24 h→用去离子水洗净后浸入由 $CaCl_2$、$NaH_2PO_4$ 和 $NaHCO_3$ 配成的过饱和钙磷溶液中，在 37 ℃水浴摇床中进行沉积 24 h 以获得涂层。为了确定 SCS 溶液的最佳配比，我先后调配了 8 种不同浓度的 SCS 溶液，最后发现当 $CaCl_2$、$NaH_2PO_4$ 和 $NaHCO_3$ 的摩尔分数分别为 5 mmol/L、2 mmol/L 和 1.5 mmol/L 时，沉积效果最好。采用这个工艺我成功地在一块尺寸为 10 mm×10 mm×2 mm 的小片钛试样上沉积了厚度大约为几十微米的羟基磷灰石涂层。

在取得了这个进展之后，我告知了中国人民解放军总医院眼科负责该项目的马骁博士。她得知这个消息后很高兴，很快就给我送来了 40 个实际使用的钛支架，希望我能用同样的工艺在这些支架表面沉积羟基磷灰石涂层。在看到这些钛支架后，我意识到一个技术难题：与形状简单的小片钛试样不同，这些钛支架大约只有 0.1 mm 厚且表面形状复杂，在不到 1 cm$^2$ 的面积上有 4 个孔。这样的几何形状给工艺中的第一步——砂纸打磨造成了极大的困难。首先，这么薄的样品本身就很难用手按着去打磨；其次，支架很可能会在打磨过程中发生塑性变形而报废。由于砂纸打磨作为提高样品表面粗糙度的步骤对于涂层沉积非常重要，因此如果这个问题无法妥善解决的话，原来的工艺将无法使用。

在查阅了更多的文献之后，我发现一篇 1998 年发表在 *Journal of Materials Science：Materials in Medicine* 上的文章中，提到可以通过一种酸碱两步法处理钛材料表面，使其易于涂层沉积[1]。根据这篇文章提供的思路，我尝试改进了原工艺：先对样品进行丙酮、乙醇、去离子水依次清洗，然后在一种混合酸 [48%$H_2SO_4$（100 ml）+18%HCl（100 ml）] 中处理 1 h，再浸入 0.6 mol/L 的 NaOH 溶液中于 160 ℃下处理 24 h，最后在 SCS 溶液中水浴沉积。酸处理是工艺改进中最核心的一环：混合酸的腐蚀作用使材料表面产生大量凹点和槽沟，在不对材料进行砂纸打磨的情况下同样提高了材料表面粗糙度。运用这个改进后的工艺，我成功地在实际使用的钛支架上沉积了羟基磷灰石涂层。图 3.1 所示为利用电子显微镜获得的涂层表面形貌以及断面形貌照片。可以看到，呈片层状的羟基磷灰石涂层在钛材料表面生长均匀，涂层厚度约为 30 μm。

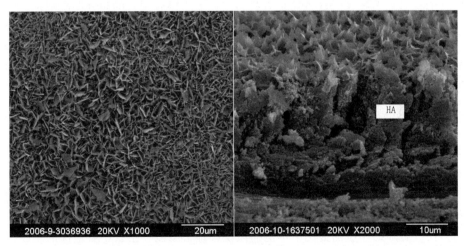

图 3.1　利用改进后的工艺在钛材料表面沉积的羟基磷灰石涂层的表面形貌以及断面形貌[2]

我向崔老师汇报了这个结果，他立即安排我在组会上向大家详细讲述整个工作。能够向硕士、博士学长们做报告，对我这个本科生而言是一次非常难得的机会。记得组会是在某个周一晚上的系会议室里开的，我的报告时间大约是 30 min。这是我第一次做科学报告，但我准备得很充分，以讲故事的口吻把遇到的技术难题以及如何巧妙解决问题的过程娓娓道来。报告得到了老师、学生们的一致好评，至今我还记得崔老师当时在听我的报告时的满面笑容，和他平时对学生一贯严厉的形象形成了鲜明对比。这是对我科研能力及表达能力的极大肯定，以至于后来我在国际学术会议上做报告时总是对自己充满信心。

中国人民解放军总医院合作方在得知我们已经成功在钛支架上生长涂层后也非常高兴。在后续实验中，马骁博士对带羟基磷灰石涂层的钛支架（HA-Ti）与不带涂层的钛支架（Ti）分别进行了体外细胞接种实验以及动物体内植入实验。细胞接种实验结果表明，HA-Ti 支架对于细胞的黏附能力远远优于作为对照组的 Ti 支架。在将这两组钛支架植入新西兰兔眼角膜基质 12 周后观测发现，HA-Ti 支架表面有大量的角膜细胞外基质黏附，材料/组织界面愈合良好；而作为对照组的 Ti 支架表面的角膜细胞仅为简单贴附，材料/组织界面没有真正愈合。这些结果表明，仿生法制备的羟基磷灰石涂层的确能够有效提高钛支架的生物活性。我非常高兴自己圆满完成了崔老师交给我的任务，也算为清华大学长了脸。这里还有一个小插曲，在大四下半学期，我的视力莫名其妙出现了下降，到北京的其他医院都看不出名堂。情急之下，我给中国人民解放军总医院的马骁博士打了电话，她不但亲自先给我查了瞳孔、眼底，还替我联系了眼科黄一飞主任的门诊，发现只是由于疲劳引起的短暂视力下降。最后由经验丰富的王丽强副主任医师替我在眼皮下进行了针对性的药物注射，不久后我的视力成功恢复。这可算是对我参与该人工角膜项目的额外奖励吧。

2006 年秋季学期开始后，我向崔老师提出了把这个工艺撰写成文章的愿望。一方面我认为这个工艺改进有一定的创新而值得发表，另一方面当时大四的我正在申请国外博士，发表文章也许能够加强自己的申请材料。一开始我想把文章投到一些国外大牌期刊，不过，崔老师认为这个工作的创新性还是更适合在国内期刊上发表，并向我推荐了《生物骨科材料与临床研究》作为投稿期刊。我花了大约 3 周时间完成了文章的初稿，然后在 9 月底把初稿发给了崔老师。在十一长假期间，崔老师发消息让我去他家讨论这篇文章。于是我某天晚上就拜访了崔老师家。寒暄了一会儿后，崔老师把我叫到书房，用电脑打开我的文章初稿，然后逐段指出文章中的不足之处。崔老师认为文章有两点需要改进：第一，需要更加明确地强调创新点在哪；第二，对于工艺背后的科学机理，在没有辅助实验的情况下不能捕风捉影地去猜测。给我印象最深的是，当时崔老师讲着讲着忽然冒出一句："科学论文不是写小说"，让我忍俊不禁。回去之后，我又花了两周时间把文章改好了，然后投到了《生物骨科材料与临床研究》编辑部。大约 1 个月后，我收到了编辑部发来的审稿意见，在按照这些意见修改后又过了 1 个月，文章终于被接收了。文章于 2007 年 2 月正式发表，这是我第一次在学术期刊上发表文章，至今记忆犹新。大四下半学期，我继续留在崔老师组里完成了毕业设计，做了一点羟基磷灰石生物陶瓷的探索性研究，不过，毕业论文最后还是以《仿生法制备羟基磷灰石涂层用于人工角膜支架》为题。

崔老师在我申请出国读博的过程中，一直给予我莫大的帮助。不仅不厌其烦地替我提交各个学校的推荐信，而且在我最终选择的时候给了我许多宝贵的建议。去美国之后，由于那边系里缺乏相关方向的导师，所以我没有继续在生物材料领域的研究，而改做传统金属材料了。然而，在崔老师组里这一年的研究训练，让我在攻读博士以及后续工作阶段一直受益匪浅。

崔老师的学术水平很高，但让我最钦佩的还是他在学术生涯中期成功转型做生物材料，并在后来真正把实验室里的成果推向了市场，为社会做出了贡献。这种跨学科、跨领域的突破，在我见过的国内外学者中真是凤毛麟角。当前，国内外学术界普遍对杂志影响因子较为崇拜，不少科研工作者为发文章而发文章，路越走越窄。与之形成鲜明对比的是崔老师这样勇于探索交叉学科，真正把产品从无到有做出来的踏实学风。目前，我国的科技政策逐渐在向后者倾斜，而崔老师的学术路线就是我们青年学者最好的榜样。

时光荏苒，从我在崔老师组里从事生产实习及毕业设计到现在已经 9 年过去了。回想那段经历乃至清华园里的时光依然是那么美好。谨以此文，向我非常尊敬的崔老师致敬。祝您 70 大寿生日快乐，桃李满天下！

# 参考文献

［1］ Wen H B, Liu Q, de Wijn J R, et al. Preparation of bioactive microporous titanium surface by a new two-step chemical treatment ［J］. *Journal of Materials Science： Materials in Medicine*, 1998, 9 (3): 121-128.

［2］ 王乐耘，王小平，崔福斋. 钛合金经酸碱两步预处理快速沉积 HA 涂层 ［J］. 生物骨科材料与临床研究，2007, 4 (1): 49-54.

# 后　记

　　此书在筹备的过程中，崔福斋教授仍然在与博士后、研究生抓紧进行着他所负责的国家 973 项目子课题、国家自然科学基金面上项目的研究工作。崔教授将他的一生奉献给了他所热爱的生物材料科学研究。他严谨的科学态度，不忘初心的科研风骨，时刻激励着我们后辈。崔老师头脑中有很多宝贵的经验积累，同时思考重要的未知，这应该就是在不断实践着"温故而知创新"的内涵。

　　崔教授虽然年届 70，但在科研思维上仍然是年轻而活跃的。现在仍然思考着学科前沿的未知科学问题的答案，例如生物矿化中早期成核机理何时是模板控制成核，何时是先成团聚集成核等。他也还在与医学专家合作研制医学急需的诸多器械，例如发明儿童颅骨缺损的修复材料，这是困扰全球神经外科医生的难题。

　　作为崔老师的学生，我们有幸和诸多专家以及昔日同门们共同回顾过往科研工作，谈谈科研创新的心得体会，并能够整理成书，谨以此书献给崔福斋教授的 70 岁生日。

　　我们也感谢为本书做出贡献的各位资深科学家们，如为本书题书名的李恒德院士，现已 95 岁高龄，仍写了 20 多幅供我们选用；年富力强的美国两院院士 Mikos 教授为本书写了很长的文章。

　　我们希望同道们能从本书中汲取有益的营养，使自己的科学生涯青出于蓝而胜于蓝。

王秀梅　杜昶

2016 年 2 月